The Athlete's Guide to Recovery

Rest, Relax, and Restore for Peak Performance

Second Edition

SAGE ROUNTREE

ROWMAN & LITTLEFIELD
Lanham • Boulder • New York • London

Published by Rowman & Littlefield
An imprint of The Rowman & Littlefield Publishing Group, Inc.
4501 Forbes Boulevard, Suite 200, Lanham, Maryland 20706
www.rowman.com

86-90 Paul Street, London EC2A 4NE

British Library Cataloguing in Publication Information Available

Library of Congress Cataloging-in-Publication Data

Names: Rountree, Sage, 1972– author.
Title: The athlete's guide to recovery : rest, relax, and restore for peak
    performance / Sage Rountree.
Description: Second edition. | Lanham, Maryland : Rowman & Littlefield,
    2024. | Summary: "Recovery—physical and mental—is a red-hot topic, and
    the worlds of sports, technology, and commerce have all taken note. This
    second edition of The Athlete's Guide to Recovery will help readers sort
    through the hype to focus on the practices and devices that really make
    a difference in recovery and lead to peak performance"—Provided by
    publisher.
Identifiers: LCCN 2023028112 (print) | LCCN 2023028113 (ebook) | ISBN
    9781538181478 (paperback) | ISBN 9781538181485 (epub)
Subjects: LCSH: Sports injuries. | Athletes—Physiology | Physical fitness.
    | Sports medicine.
Classification: LCC RD97 .R68 2024 (print) | LCC RD97 (ebook) | DDC
    617.1/027—dc23/eng/20230905
LC record available at https://lccn.loc.gov/2023028112
LC ebook record available at https://lccn.loc.gov/2023028113

♾️ The paper used in this publication meets the minimum requirements of
American National Standard for Information Sciences—Permanence of Paper
for Printed Library Materials, ANSI/NISO Z39.48-1992.

The Athlete's Guide to Recovery

To Wes, Lillian, and Vivian

Training = stress + rest. The most important component of this equation is rest, but no one is going to get rich writing a triathlon book about rest.

—Tom Rodgers, *The Perfect Distance*

Contents

Acknowledgments

Research for this book was a joy. In the dozens of in-person, phone, Zoom, and e-mail interviews I conducted, I learned more than I could ever fit into one book. I'm deeply grateful to everyone who spoke with me, and especially to those who demonstrated how powerful working in a field you love passionately can be. For the first edition, these include, in alphabetical order, Pat Archer, Brian Beatty, Annette Bednosky, Ben Benjamin, Dave Berkoff, Gale Bernhardt, Chris Bohannon, Evie Boswell-Vilt, Jeff Brown, Gordo Byrn, Steven Cole, Bernard Condevaux, Kristen Dieffenbach, Matt Dixon, Jamie Donaldson, Andy Doyle, Charlie Engle, Reed Ferber, Shalane Flanagan, Carl Foster, Joe Friel, James Green, Kate Hays, Jeff Hunt, Gilad Jacobs, Nate Jenkins, Marc Jeuland, Leah Kangas, Jay T. Kearney, Kristin Keim, Michael Kellmann, Göran Kenttä, Nikki Kimball, Thomas Laffont, Carolyn Levy, Amanda Lovato, Peter Magill, Alex McDonald, Stephen McGregor, Greg McMillan, Tera Moody, Jack Raglin, Mike Ricci, Tom Rodgers, Hal Rosenberg, Monique Ryan, Bill Sands, Bob Seebohar, Stephen Seiler, Kami Semick, Todd Straka, Keith Straw, Jennifer Van Allen, Sue Walsh, Michael Wardian, Peter Watson, Matthew Weatherley-White, and Marv Zauderer. Matt Fitzgerald was an especially warm cheerleader in the rollout of that first edition—thank you, Matt! For this second edition, I had wonderful conversations with Sian Allen, Marco Altini, Andy Blow, Tim DeBoom, Matt Dixon, Matt Driller, Robert Furberg, Danielle Adams Norenberg, Nick Tiller, and Scott Tindal.

Thank you to the wonderful crew at Rowman & Littlefield for carrying this book into a second edition. Christen Karniski, Samantha Delwarte, copyeditor Nancy Syrett, cover designer Dustin Watson, proofreader Annette Van Deusen, and production editor Nicole Carty all helped make this edition as useful as possible for you, the reader! Thanks also to Bob Kern and Linda Konner for their agenting on the first and second editions of this work.

Thank you to my favorite people with whom to sit and do nothing: my family. My parents and my many fantastic in-laws have been my company in many happy postrace lounging hours. And thank you especially to my daughters, Lillian and Vivian, and most especially to my husband, Wes. I can think of no greater way to spend my time than relaxing with you three.

Introduction

Sports—endurance sports, in particular—are about testing the limits. You work your body to a breaking point, then step away from the brink, let the work absorb, and repeat. It sounds simple, but the process is not clear-cut. Where is that breaking point? It's a moving target, varying from athlete to athlete, year to year, month to month, and sometimes even day to day. How long does absorption take? Again, it's hard to tell. Rest too much, and you miss out on gains that could mean the difference between fulfilling your potential and falling flat. Rest too little, and you drive your performance into a downward spiral that can take days, weeks, months, or years to mitigate. The key is finding the balance between working enough and resting enough, and that's what this book will help you do. Following the recovery tools laid out here, you'll figure out how to achieve your optimal balance.

As an athlete, I've pushed the limits myself. I ran myself into—and beyond—a tibial stress fracture, and then, to avoid losing too much fitness, I spent many long "runs" churning circles in the deep end of the pool for hours on end. I overachieved on a field test to measure my lactate threshold and wound up spending a four-month block training for a marathon with my heart rate zones skewed almost 10 beats too high, so that all the work that was supposed to be performed just below my lactate threshold was actually redlining me. I've been so deep in fatigue during Ironman training that I desperately looked forward to a teeth cleaning, because I'd get to lie down in the dentist's chair. I understand how tough it can be to take the time for recovery, even when it's really in my best interest.

I spent many years coaching athletes in endurance and ultraendurance events. As a coach, I took a more objective view of recovery than I did as an athlete. Much of a coach's work is instructing athletes to take it easy, building rest days, rest weeks, and rest months into training schedules—it's as much about what not to do as what to do. I spent much more time assuring my athletes that missing a workout is okay than pushing them to get things done. From reading logs and talking to my athletes, I could see when the edges started to fray and pull their training back so they could absorb the hard work before returning to intense workouts.

As a yoga teacher, I know the benefits of rest, relaxation, lying down, and breathing. As I tell my students, going into a deep expression of a yoga pose isn't the path to enlightenment. But knowing when *not* to work deeper may help you down the path, because it shows self-awareness and an acceptance of what is going on in your body moment to moment. This self-knowledge is crucial for success in sports and in life, and you can develop it by using the recovery tools outlined in this book. Some of them come from yoga, many more come from sports science, and all of them are proven time and again in athletes' bodies. Best of all, the most effective and valuable recovery methods are free.

Since the first edition of this book came out in 2011, we've seen an enhanced attention to the importance of recovery—and the COVID-19 pandemic has shifted our relationship to rest in interesting ways. It both forced us to slow down and, for many, upended daily routines in ways that will continue to reverberate for years. Wearable technology and social media have also exploded since 2011, so that athletes now must wade through a lot of noise about data points and gimmicky recovery tools to find what will work for them. Consider that photos of ice baths are exciting. Pictures of someone sleeping are not. I hope this second edition will help you keep your focus on the tested and proved recovery tools that will enhance not only your training and performance but also your overall health and energy.

While my experience and the focus of this book are mainly endurance sports, if you are a team sports player, you will also find actionable advice here. This book gives you the tools for learning about your own body and its optimal conditions for recovery, so that you can reach peak performance while feeling balanced and content with your sport and your life. In part I, we'll examine the psychological and physiological processes involved in recovery to see its vital importance in training, and we'll see what can go wrong when recovery is insufficient and an athlete moves into overtraining. You'll learn ways to measure your own state of recovery, both qualitatively and quantitatively, and we'll look at some general guidelines for returning to training after injury or illness.

Part II gives you concrete, proven techniques to enhance your recovery and improve performance. They cover everything from stress-reduction tips to nutrition and supplements to technological aids and massage. (The secret: There is no secret! Attention to the fundamentals will get you farther than any hot new product.) You'll also learn some very simple poses, breathing exercises, and meditation techniques to enhance your recovery and your overall health.

Finally, part III shows you how to put it all together, demonstrating various plans for recovery from training for and competing in events of all types, from short-distance bike races to ultramarathons. These chapters will give you a starting point from which to develop your own routines, based on how your body responds to the various techniques. Using the modalities described here, you'll improve the speed and quality of your recovery, hit peak performance, and grow more balanced, happy, and successful in your sport and your life.

Part I

DEFINING AND MEASURING RECOVERY

1

Why Recovery Matters

To do nothing is sometimes a good remedy.

—*Hippocrates*

In summer 2009, I spent a week in residence at the Olympic Training Center (OTC) in Colorado Springs, enjoying a coaching internship with USA Triathlon. It was exciting to see the resources we give our most elite athletes. The training center offers a full-featured training facility, with all the amenities you might expect: full rooms of weight training equipment, ample gyms (I taught yoga in a roomy tae kwon do space, outfitted with lovely cushioned mats), indoor and outdoor pools, and a cafeteria serving healthy food and drinks. Miles of local trails and roads, including some that head right up into the Rockies, make this a fantastic place to train. Better still, the OTC boasts a Recovery Center. This luxe facility, available to all resident athletes, includes a steam room, a sauna, a hot tub, a cold plunge pool, a snack bar, and rooms for yoga and massage. The USA Triathlon national team members are allotted 90 minutes of massage time a week, which they can use at one session or divide into multiple, shorter sessions. In a convenient central location on the training center campus, the Recovery Center puts at athletes' fingertips the best recovery modalities known to sports scientists.

At the Olympic team level, athletes know the importance both of managing every element important to training and of prioritizing recovery. Remember, Olympians and other elite athletes are not operating on five hours of sleep, squeezing in their workouts in the early-morning dark before sitting around conference room tables or chasing children around all day. Nor are they wrapping up evening workouts after a long day at the office in time to mow the lawn before daylight fades. Between workouts, they rest.

Although it's probably unrealistic for you to prioritize your recovery to such an extent, if you can give a fraction of this value to your own recovery, your performance will improve. Perhaps not to Olympic levels, but certainly in ways that will convince you of the importance and benefit of rest. Recovery is where the gains of your training actually occur, and valuing your recovery is the key to both short-term and long-term success, no matter what your sport.

Any attention that you can give to your recovery is likely to be helpful. One study of British rugby players measuring the effectiveness of active recovery, compression garments, and contrast baths found they were all more useful than doing nothing.[1] By choosing to do one thing to enhance your recovery, you are probably more likely to do more, creating a positive spiral.

In this book, we'll consider various ways to describe, measure, and enhance recovery between bouts of training and competing. Recovery is a complicated and emerging field, and much of the research on these recovery techniques is still preliminary and even contradictory. Some techniques will work wonders for you; others won't. Ultimately, you'll need to be an experiment of one person, learning what works best for you.

THE WORK/REST CYCLE

Life moves in a cyclical pattern. We see it all around us in the natural world: As the earth travels around the sun, the seasons shift. As the moon travels around the earth, the amount of its lit surface visible to us changes. As the earth rotates on its axis, day and night alternate.

Our bodies move through cycles, too. The aging process that takes us from birth to death is the broadest, but we echo nature's cycles as well—especially if we engage in seasonal sports or target a peak race once or twice a year. We cycle through the course of an athletic career, through annual training plans (which we call macrocycles), through smaller blocks of training (mesocycles), through the workouts in a week (microcycles), and through periods of activity and inactivity each day. These cycles depend not only on the periods in which we work but also on the periods in which we rest and build our recovery. It's the balance between the work and the rest that keeps us healthy and strong.

This balancing act is described by Carl Weigert's law of supercompensation, formulated in the late 19th century, and by Hans Selye's general adaptation syndrome. An endocrinologist working in the mid-20th century, Selye identified two kinds of stress: positive stress, called "eustress," and negative stress, called "distress." We adapt to the former—indeed, it's important for our growth—but when we do not, the stress changes into the latter, with physiological consequences. While we may do better under pressure, too much pressure quickly becomes a problem. We travel from the alarm stage, in which stress hormones are released to allow the body to respond to the stressor; to the resistance stage, in which the body works to bring itself back into balance by adapting; and, finally, into the exhaustion stage, in which continued stress leads to hormonal imbalance and changes to the chemistry of the tissues can lead to illness and even death. Figure 1.1 illustrates this progression.

What prevents us from moving into this exhaustion stage? Recovery. When we manage stress and take time to adapt to stress stimuli, our bodies undergo positive changes that equip us to handle the stressors we face. These adaptations are called "supercompensation." During this process, the tissues in the body undergo change in response to the stress put on them. Ultimately, they become better able to cope with the stressor. This happens in four phases,[2] illustrated in figure 1.2.

In the first phase of supercompensation, which encompasses the hour or two immediately following an intense workout, fatigue is high.

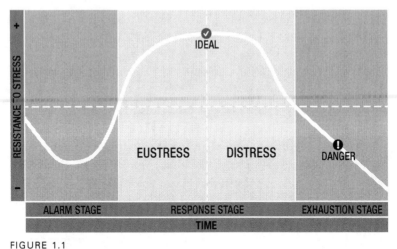

FIGURE 1.1
General adaptation syndrome
Note: Positive stress can turn into negative stress without adaptation.

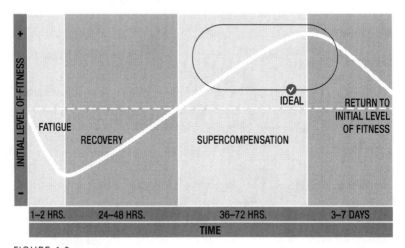

FIGURE 1.2
Phases of adaptation
Note: Time your next hard workout to rebound off your supercompensation from the previous one.

It comes from reduced neural activation, depleted muscle glycogen stores, and mental fatigue related to serotonin levels in the brain. Cortisol levels are high as the sympathetic nervous system (the fight-or-flight response) dominates. The body is compromised on a neural and psychological level, and it needs rest. The athlete feels spent and perhaps a little mentally fuzzy.

The second phase of supercompensation comprises one to two days following the workout. During this period, the body begins to recover. The body's energy stores of adenosine triphosphate (ATP) and muscle glycogen are replenished. This happens very quickly in the case of ATP and more slowly for muscle glycogen, depending on how long the exercise lasted and how well the athlete refueled during and immediately after the workout. The body consumes more oxygen, a process known as excess postexercise oxygen consumption (EPOC), and it uses more energy even at rest, as it works to restore protein and balance hormones.

In the third phase after a workout, somewhere between 36 and 72 hours later, the adaptive gains occur. The body has adapted, which the athlete can experience both physically in a renewed ability to generate force and mentally in a sense of confidence and readiness to train. This is the stage in which the next training stimulus should be applied to take advantage of this freshness and build on it.

If you miss this window and pass into stage 4 of supercompensation, which includes days 3 to 7 after the initial workout, the body will begin to return to its original state, and the adaptations effected in the previous stages will be lost. Thus, the trick to successful training lies in properly timing the frequency and intensity of workouts. You'll be able to do so only when you have a sense of whether you are recovered enough for another hard session. That's the subject of this book: how to get there and how to know you're there.

Managing your cycle of supercompensation requires awareness of your short-term recovery (that is, how you respond to an individual workout), but training usually involves a series of workouts, some more critical than others. You'll need to be sure that you're not undermining your body's adaptation by working too hard in the interim periods between your key workouts. You also need to apply the proper training stimulus: If your load is correct and your recovery is correct, you'll adapt. If your load is insufficient, you'll plateau. And if your load is too heavy for your recovery, your performance will suffer, and you risk overtraining. Proper training stimulus varies according to your age, experience, background, and a host of other factors; you'll learn it by trial and error, and a coach can be a valuable partner. Coaches can also ensure you're taking proper recovery.

Recovery involves more than just the physiological or neurochemical processes at work. It also requires psychological restoration, or a renewed desire to train. Without this sense of enjoyment, your sport will not be a healthy part of your life. You'll gain this sense of restoration by including rest in your daily, weekly, monthly, and annual cycles.

Part of the mystery of recovery is exactly how to define it. Is recovery supercompensation, or is it a return to the baseline? Is recovery muscle adaptation? Is recovery readiness to train, and, if so, how can we be sure an athlete's perceived readiness is in alignment with their ability to perform? Ultimately, it's tough to pinpoint exactly what recovery means, and precisely when it happens. We know when we are not recovered, because our results are worse than expected and we don't feel well in training and competition. Thus good performance will be your indication of sufficient recovery.

RECOVERY OVER TIME

Recovery takes place in both the short term and the long term. Short-term recovery follows from paying attention to your rest and recuperation day to day. Long-term recovery comes from good short-term recovery and from giving your body adequate time to recover between your peak efforts. Here's how recovery should cycle through your day, week, month, and year.

In a Day

You recover during the course of the day by alternating the amount of time you spend in training activities with down time. It can include passive rest and sleep, but you'll also be recovering even as you go about your daily activities. Your body is processing your meals to rebuild your muscles and restore your glycogen supply; it is managing inflammation; it is, holistically, enjoying the cycle between work and rest.

There should also be periods of mental rest built into your day. If you move from sleep right into a workout, from a workout right into work, from work into meetings, and from meetings into chores, you don't get any mental downtime. Be sure you take a few brain breaks to stare out the window; to go for an easy walk away from computer, phone, and TV screens; or to talk to a friend. Any enjoyable activity is fine, provided it's relaxing and not associated with training or work.

In a Week

During the course of your week, or microcycle, recovery comes in the cyclical pattern of harder and easier workout days. On the hard days, workouts targeting strength and power and taxing the aerobic and anaerobic systems push the boundaries of what an athlete can do. The easier days are the key here: They must be quite easy, to give your body time to recover and adapt to the stressors you've placed on it. All too often, athletes gravitate toward the mushy middle, between working easy enough for recovery and hard enough to target lactate threshold, VO_2max, neuromuscular efficiency, or power. This leaves them too tired to perform at their best in their harder workouts, robbing them of the chance to eke out a slightly faster pace or slightly higher wattage and to improve speed and power.

The big question, then, is how best to alternate hard and easy days. The big answer is this: It depends. A range of factors will affect the answer: your age, the impact level of the sport, your history in the sport and any past or present injuries, environmental factors during workouts, the length of your race, and, ultimately, how well you recover. Here are various examples. In tables 1.1 and 1.2, hard/easy days alternate. For a masters athlete, or one new to the sport, two hard days a week might suffice.

Table 1.1. Hard/easy alternation

MONDAY	TUESDAY	WEDNESDAY	THURSDAY	FRIDAY	SATURDAY	SUNDAY
Off	Hard	Easy	Hard	Easy	Hard	Easy

Table 1.2. Hard/easy alternation for a masters or novice athlete

MONDAY	TUESDAY	WEDNESDAY	THURSDAY	FRIDAY	SATURDAY	SUNDAY
Off	Hard	Easy	Easy	Hard	Easy	Easy

Of course, these schedules do not include moderate workouts, which do have their place (see table 1.3).

Table 1.3. Hard/easy/moderate alternation

MONDAY	TUESDAY	WEDNESDAY	THURSDAY	FRIDAY	SATURDAY	SUNDAY
Off	Hard	Easy	Moderate	Easy	Hard	Easy

For those who can tolerate more frequent hard workouts (for example, in nonimpact sports), two hard days can go back to back (see table 1.4).

Table 1.4. Hard/hard/easy alternation

MONDAY	TUESDAY	WEDNESDAY	THURSDAY	FRIDAY	SATURDAY	SUNDAY
Off	Hard	Hard	Easy	Easy	Hard	Easy

Or, if you want two hard days in a row but also want to include some moderate work, you could try the schedule in table 1.5.

Table 1.5. Hard/hard/easy/moderate alternation

MONDAY	TUESDAY	WEDNESDAY	THURSDAY	FRIDAY	SATURDAY	SUNDAY
Off	Hard	Hard	Easy	Moderate	Hard	Easy

In a Month

Your training mesocycle lasts approximately a month. These meso-cycles usually follow a 3 to 1 work/rest ratio, with 2 to 1 a standard ap-proach for masters athletes. In these ratios, each microcycle emphasizes either work (3 or 2 microcycles) or rest (1 microcycle). Each mesocycle should contain a contiguous block of easier days to allow you to absorb and adapt to the work of the preceding weeks. For most athletes, this takes the form of an easy week, though some experienced and elite ath-letes will step back for a shorter block of around five days (which leaves the weekends for heavier training, often with a group). During your easy, "rest," or stepback week, your workouts should scale back in terms of both duration and intensity—and possibly also frequency. Thus your workouts would be shorter and carry less, if any, intensity, and you might drop one or two workouts in the stepback week.

This week is often used for fitness testing, especially in coach Joe Fri-el's approach to training, outlined in the *Training Bible* books.[3] Testing provides a valuable opportunity to measure your progress and check the state of your recovery. As we'll see in chapter 2, declines in performance are an early sign of overtraining. Make sure, however, that you aren't testing to the detriment of your resting. Even when you have some field tests in your stepback week, you should leave the week feeling fresher than when you went in.

This freshness is key. During each month, your cumulative fatigue will mount, even as you include recovery for supercompensation. The rest week in your cycle lets the fatigue lift and long-term adaptation oc-cur, so that you can be fresher as you start the next mesocycle. Figures 1.3 and 1.4 demonstrate typical mesocycle builds as well as the amount of fatigue and freshness an athlete carries through the cycle.

Note that while you might want to schedule a rest week during a period of heavier stress at work, travel, or family obligations, that isn't a wise approach. Cumulative stress will make that just another week where you didn't recover. Be wise in scheduling your rest weeks, and be proactive in taking an unscheduled rest week, or half a rest week,

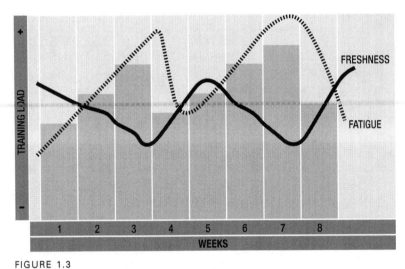

FIGURE 1.3
Mesocycle of 3 to 1
Note: Freshness falls and fatigue builds over the mesocycle; recovery weeks reverse the trend.

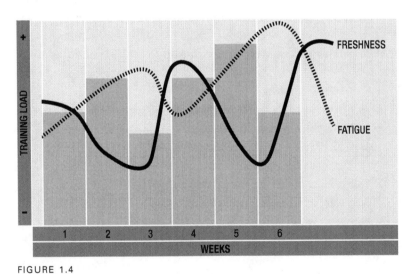

FIGURE 1.4
Mesocycle of 2 to 1
Note: A 2-to-1 mesocycle works well for newer or older athletes.

because you feel you need it. This can be the proverbial stitch that, in time, saves nine.

In a Season or Year

Just as it appears in the day, week, and month, cyclicality applies during the course of your year. Be sure to block out time each season or year when you turn your focus away from organized training. You can and should be active during this period, but your activity should be varied and fun and completely free of the attention to the parameters you control during your main sport training. As you chart your time spent in training during the year, you should see definite peaks and valleys. These valleys are important, as they allow you time to recover from the rigors of training, both physically and mentally.

Beyond this annual variability, there may even be periods where you push for a few years, then step back to focus on a shorter distance or to train less, perhaps in conjunction with other obligations in your family or work life. Olympic athletes follow a four-year cycle. Yours might be shorter—training harder for two years and stepping back, or going for a sabbatical, a lighter year, every seven years. It need not be a planned step back; your life circumstances will often dictate when it is time to go lighter. Thus the cycle plays out on a grand level.

VALUING RECOVERY

To receive the benefits of recovery—and hence, to get the most out of your training—you must pay as much attention to recovery as you do to your training. That means treating recovery as an extension of your training, which it is, and approaching it with the same zeal. You have to go easy to be able to go hard. Exercise physiologist Carl Foster says athletes must "be disciplined enough and prepare hard enough for training, which means you sometimes have to do very little. Yoga, icing, meditation, massage: work as hard at that as running your 20-mile run."

Attention to recovery might take even more discipline than training. Two-time Ironman® world champion Tim DeBoom said to me in 2010 that, after his many years in triathlon, "Training has become the easy part. All the supplemental exercises, stretches, and therapies are what make the difference now." Ultrarunner Charlie Engle agrees. "The easiest thing for me to do any given day is to run out the door," he says. "The hardest thing to do is all these other things that will actually help keep me healthy through the years." Foster, who has worked with U.S. Speedskating, remembers that Bonnie Blair and Dan Jansen focused on their recovery so much they called themselves the No Fun Guys. Foster explains, "When you're a full-time athlete, it's actually amazingly boring. A lot of people with physical talent drop out of it because the lifestyle is too constraining. You have to have the discipline to be one of the No Fun Guys—and that's no fun."

Paying attention to recovery not only can be tough but also can run counter to the athletic mind-set. As athletes, we are familiar with the intensity of work, comfortable with suffering, and often unreasonably proud of our ability to handle more, more, more. But Engle cautions that the body needs to balance work with recovery. "You can drive your car across the country and then get in the car and drive the next day. You can't do the same thing with the body," he says. "There's a weird badge of honor that if you ran a marathon, you can get up and run the next day. People forget that you have to rest."

That amnesia ties in to a cultural sense that action is the only way to achieve results. There is no room for passive downtime in this worldview. Sport performance coach and psychotherapist Marv Zauderer says, "In Western culture, we tend to be consumed by the perspective that the thing that we want to happen—getting stronger, faster, fitter—is happening only when we're working on it, exerting some kind of control. We aren't used to the idea that letting go, resting, and relaxing control can be as important to healing, recovery, and strengthening as they are."

In our hyperbusy culture, it can be hard to be still. Often, a planned rest day devolves into a day of housework, and a rest week becomes a week of playing catch-up at work. Whenever possible, dial back and delegate. Use your energy where it is best spent. Ultrarunner Keith Straw suggests you avoid your chores. "When you rest, *rest*," he says. "Don't rake the leaves, don't clean the gutters." Athletic therapist Reed Ferber says, "A rest day is working nothing but your thumb on the remote control."

Ultrarunner and sports scientist Nick Tiller says that, while many athletes shy away from taking even a single rest day, "I've always been an advocate of rest days and easy weeks. For me, personally, every fifth or sixth week, I try to reduce my training volume and just get my body time to adapt—particularly when I'm running ultras. I might even just take a week off from running and do no running at all. You're not really going to lose a great deal of fitness or endurance in five, six, seven days of inactivity. Any more than that, you want to be careful, but when you return you're going to be [in] much better shape. After all, training doesn't make you fitter: *recovering* from training does." This points to some of the strongest skills to hone for your recovery: patience and faith.

PATIENCE AND FAITH

Your successful approach to recovery will depend on two traits: patience and faith. You need patience so that you can give your body the time it needs to heal itself. Your body is an amazing, complicated, and powerful system, and given time, it will adapt in incredible ways to the stresses you put on it. But you have to give it time.

Faith is also crucial. You need to trust that time off, even though it might be hard to take, will have a direct, positive effect on your training. In time, you'll see that it does, and your faith will become a tested and proven belief. Patience and faith are heightened by the power of ritual. Simply taking the time to sit in a warm bath or to practice restorative yoga sends the very powerful signal that you value your recovery enough to work on it. When you regularly go through the steps of your recovery protocol, you'll be ingraining positive habits, and the pattern of taking these steps will signal to your parasympathetic nervous system that it's time to relax, to restore, to recover.

It's also okay to put your faith in the modalities that you enjoy or find appealing, whether or not there's hard evidence that they work. Sports scientist Sian Allen says: "As long as there are no obvious negative effects, the best form of recovery might often be the one you actually enjoy doing and so can commit to making a habit, or believe it's working for you. The placebo effect can often be dismissed or underrated, but there are some viable mechanisms there!" If you have the time and means to enjoy a recovery tool that hasn't been proven harmful, go for it. Any attention to recovery adds to your net gain.

2

Avoiding Overtraining

Now that we've looked at the recovery cycle and its benefits, let's investigate what happens when you don't recover. Under-recovery is a slippery slope that can lead to full-blown overtraining syndrome. Overtraining is a specter that looms just over the hill of most dedicated athletes' training, but it is a mysterious state that is hard, if not impossible, to diagnose, with both physiological and psychological implications. This amorphousness has been combined with confusing terminology that calls overtraining "staleness," "burnout," or "overwork." Sometimes overtraining is described as an imbalance between training and rest; sometimes it is described, more holistically, as an imbalance between *stress* and rest. This latter definition includes all the life stressors that combine with training stressors and contribute to problems in the athlete who does not allow for recovery.

It's useful to think of overtraining as one point on a spectrum (figure 2.1)—the training equivalent to exhaustion, the third stage of Hans Selye's stress adaptation chart. Before an athlete progresses into overtraining, he moves further along the spectrum. When we apply an increasingly stressful training load, we go into a period of intentional overreaching, which involves carrying a heavy load for a week or two, then pulling back and absorbing the work by devoting adequate time and attention to recovery. It's pushing the body to the brink and then

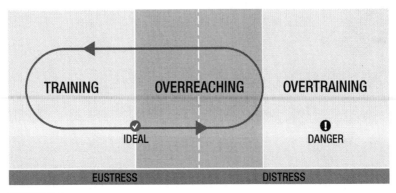

FIGURE 2.1
Training response spectrum

yanking back before the athlete topples over the edge. A powerful and useful strategy for training, overreaching happens notably at training camps of a week or 10 days' length.

Such stress must be followed, of course, by sufficient recovery. An athlete will leave a period of intentional overreaching with a large load of fatigue. That should be enough to generate positive adaptations through supercompensation, without pushing the athlete into injury or illness. Kristen Dieffenbach, executive director of the United States Center for Coaching Excellence, likens the work of overreaching to getting just the right toast on a marshmallow. You need to come close to the fire (a heavy training stimulus) to create change in the marshmallow (the body). "You want it to be brown and crinkly, without catching on fire," she says. "How it comes out depends on how hot the fire is, and where you're standing."

The fine line between perfectly roasting the marshmallow and incinerating it needs special attention. You must know when to pull back from the fire and cool off. Coach Gordo Byrn, endurance coach and co-author of *Going Long*, explains, "There are times when it's desirable to get pretty tired. But you need to prepare for those overload periods and bear in mind that they're special occasions. Athletes get trapped in this idea that they need to be exhausted to improve." The success of your overreaching period, Byrn explains, has less to do with the numbers you can post during the week and more to do with how well—and how quickly—you can recover from the overload.

This ability to recover quickly is key, and it can save you from progressing further along the spectrum toward full overtraining. When you are carrying big fatigue, you should be able to rebound after a few days of rest or very light training. This pre-overtraining state is characterized by a performance decline. Keeping a detailed training log and regularly testing your performance in the field can alert you if such a decline begins. Next come feelings of fatigue that feel like "dead legs." As alarming as this may sound, it isn't full-blown overtraining; careful attention to rest can still avert the shift toward a more serious problem.

But if the load is too great, for too long, or if your training is too monotonous, including too much of the same stimulus day in and day out, and if your recovery continues to be insufficient, you can bring yourself into a state of overtraining.

HOW TO IDENTIFY OVERTRAINING
Psychological indicators often point to a state of overtraining sooner and more clearly than do physiological indicators, such as blood tests and heart rate measurements. Because psychological and physiological issues such as depression and thyroid problems can resemble overtraining, it's important to work with an experienced health care practitioner to make the appropriate diagnosis.

Signs of overtraining can be nebulous. An overtrained athlete may exhibit a cluster of the symptoms listed below while not showing others. And because many of these symptoms can indicate other underlying medical conditions, do not use this list as a self-diagnostic tool. Instead, consult with your coach and health care providers.

Psychological Indicators of Overtraining
- Loss of interest in competition and training
- Loss of ability to focus, both in training and at work

- Loss of appetite
- Lower sex drive
- Loss of sleep
- Clumsiness
- Bad mood
- Irritability

Physiological Indicators of Overtraining
- Decline in performance
- Heavy, lifeless, "dead" feeling in the legs
- Weight loss
- Gauntness
- Thirst
- Raised heart rate at rest, during postural shifts, and/or after exercise
- Dizziness
- Muscle soreness that does not abate
- Swollen lymph nodes
- Gastrointestinal (GI) trouble, especially diarrhea
- Frequent illness
- Slow healing
- Amenorrhea (loss of menstrual period)

Thinking about overtraining continues to change, but most agree that it's reversible only by a prolonged period of rest, one that can last for weeks or even months. Hence, your athletic success depends on purposely avoiding pushing yourself into such a state.

RED-S and the Female Athlete Triad

A gender-nonspecific condition, relative energy deficiency in sport, or RED-S, is a state in which the demands an athlete places on their body outweigh the energy they are taking in. This can coincide with disordered eating, in which an athlete doesn't consume enough fuel to power their workouts, and/or with training that outpaces the available energy—i.e., one way to define overtraining. RED-S overlaps in great part with the Female Athlete Triad, a cluster of three conditions: low energy availability, amenorrhea, and low bone density. The term *RED-S* was coined by the International Olympic Committee in 2014 and as such is relatively new, so not only might your health care team not know to screen you for this issue, but they may not be familiar with the terminology. Advocate for yourself if you feel you may suffer from RED-S. There's a useful information page at red-s.com with a screening quiz and resources for athletes. Much of what you'll learn about in this book—tools for sleeping well, managing stress, and feeding to fuel your training—will complement medical advice if you are battling RED-S.

HOW TO PREVENT OVERTRAINING

This book examines the many practical things you can do to prevent overtraining: focus on your recovery nutrition; make sleep a priority; find a balance among training, work, and relationships; and employ recovery strategies such as wearing compression clothing and practicing restorative yoga. On the broadest level, though, simply knowing your goals and paying close attention to your body will help keep you from overtraining.

Context is everything. Setting appropriate goals and keeping the big picture in mind throughout the season will help athletes stay away from overtraining. Sport performance coach and psychotherapist Marv Zauderer says that overtraining is a common result of an athlete setting unrealistic goals. If you have set your goal so high that it becomes all-consuming, then you're going to take a hit, and that can easily move you into overtraining. In addition, anxiety often causes athletes to seek to exert control. When athletes feel anxious, Zauderer says, they turn to the things they think they can control—for example, the volume and intensity of their training—often to the detriment of their recovery.

Carl Foster, professor emeritus of exercise physiology at the University of Wisconsin–La Crosse, agrees that the problem is a need for control. In his years working at a teaching hospital, he says, "I'd see the residents, tired all the time, do boneheaded things that don't have good outcomes. Then did they go home and sleep? No, they'd go to the library and read up on the issues. Similarly, if artistic performers have a less than stellar performance, they do more rehearsal." An accomplishment-oriented mind-set causes the trouble, Foster explains. "That's how you get over-training syndrome. You say, 'I'm out of shape, I need to work harder,'" when you're not out of shape at all; you're simply unrested.

Paying attention to your psychological and physiological states is key. Know your habits, know your stressors, and know your goals. Beyond that self-awareness, keep careful track of your performance in workouts and races and analyze it to confirm that you are adapting as planned. A decline in performance should lead to a search for its cause and to a focus on the quality of your recovery. Remember, often doing less is more powerful than training more.

In chapters 3 and 4, we'll look at ways to qualify and quantify the state of your recovery. Tracking metrics such as mood, hours slept, and various physiological parameters will help you keep an eye on the state of your recovery and hence your training. Best of all, they will help you calibrate your innate internal sense of whether you are ready for more work. Such attentiveness will keep you from approaching a state of overtraining as well as help you reach your peak potential.

QUICK TIPS

- Overtraining is a serious condition from which it can take months to recover. Pay attention to the state of your recovery so that you don't reach an overtrained state.
- Taking a few days off at the first sign of under-recovery can yank you back from the edge.
- The signs of overtraining can also be symptoms of other medical conditions, including RED-S; check with your health care provider.
- Sometimes doing less is far more powerful than doing more.

3

Qualitative Measurements of Recovery

Think about the last time you felt really refreshed. (Hopefully, it's not too distant a memory.) What adjectives would you use to describe the feeling? You might use words like *springy*, *peppy*, or *on*, as in, "I felt *on* today." The vocabulary will differ from athlete to athlete, and you shouldn't feel surprised if it's tough to put words to the feeling of recovery. Since recovery is a broad and somewhat nebulous state, it can be very hard to identify. Often it is defined more by its absence than by its presence. While there are some ways to quantify recovery—and we'll look at them in chapter 4—you will be best served by taking a qualitative impression of your state of recovery. This is an important way to pick up on early warning signs that can't be quantified. Exercise physiologist Stephen Seiler, a professor at the University of Agder in Norway, says, "Perceptual and psychological measures are more useful for picking up a tendency toward overreaching states than quantitative measures like blood tests, heart rate variability, et cetera. By the time those variables paint a clear picture, the athlete is often already in trouble." Thus you're wise to stay attuned to how you feel day to day, and to find words to describe and track this feeling.

Stephen McGregor developed the running Training Stress Score (rTSS) in WKO+, a method of quantifying recovery (see chapter 4).

But McGregor sees measuring recovery as both a science and an art. He says, "I think of coaching a bit like medicine. There's a scientific aspect to medicine, but we still need doctors with intuition to qualitatively evaluate the information. The quantitative tools give you information, objectivity, baseline data, and at the end of the day it comes back to the intuition." Honing your intuition and assessment skills will help you keep an accurate eye on your fatigue level.

Ultrarunner Michael Wardian, who has placed third overall at the Marathon des Sables, a six-day, 151-mile race in the Sahara, likens his awareness of his recovery to a car checkup. When his legs feel dead, that reads like low tire pressure and is a sign to change his workout schedule accordingly. His self-assessment is like a systems check: "Is my tank fueled? Is the engine feeling good? How about the tires? What are my gauges showing?"

For a visual aid in this tracking, use a training log. Your training log is a tool to help you calibrate, to learn how to tune in to your body. After a period of using it regularly, you might be able to work more on intuition. Consider this analogy: As you begin endurance sports training, you go on feel, working at levels that feel sustainable for longer workouts, or pushing during shorter ones. After a few blow-ups in which you push too hard, you learn about your current limits. Then you might begin training with a heart rate monitor, GPS, or power meter. Training with this device reduces the guesswork, removing the trial and error. You get to know when you might push a little more, or when you're in danger of being forced to slow down. Eventually, you'll develop a sense of what your heart rate, speed, or wattage is at a given effort, and you may ultimately stop using the monitor for some or even all of your workouts. You've been calibrated, and you've had your intuitive sense of effort and pacing confirmed. Keeping your log is like wearing that heart rate monitor, or using a GPS or power meter: It helps you see the patterns. It gives you some gauges so that you can see into the state of the system. In time, you may choose to operate more on feel.

INVENTORIES TO MEASURE RECOVERY

Various inventories and lists have been scientifically proven to track recovery. Professor Jack Raglin, a sport psychologist at Indiana University, explains that these inventories work just as well as any physiological measurement of recovery. "Whatever logical or theoretically compelling physiological assessment you look at, these correlate with psychological measures," he says. "How you feel is a reflection of what's going on."

Coaches and sports psychologists have noted that the Profile of Mood States (POMS) questionnaire developed by Douglas McNair and his colleagues[1] can predict whether an athlete is well rested or overtrained. This scale measures six mood states: tension, depression, anger, vigor, fatigue, and confusion. Obviously, one of these things is not like the other: vigor. In a well-rested athlete, a graph of the POMS profile will peak for vigor while showing lower scores in the other five states. It is called the "iceberg profile," for its jutting top. In an under-recovered or overtrained athlete, the opposite occurs.

Building on the POMS, Michael Kellmann and Wolfgang Kallus developed a questionnaire to track athletes' stress and recovery, the Recovery-Stress Questionnaire for Athletes, or RESTQ-Sport.[2] This 72-item questionnaire asks athletes to rank both the stress they are experiencing and how recovered they feel. The stress questions track markers of general, emotional, and social stress (conflicts/pressure, fatigue, lack of energy, and physical complaints), as well as rest intervals, halftimes, and time-outs; emotional exhaustion; and injury. Recovery questions track success; social and physical recovery; well-being; sleep quality; and the sense of being in shape, personal accomplishment, self-efficacy, and self-regulation. There is also an abbreviated 36-question version that seems to work well.[3]

This thorough tool, used in national programs, is not officially available online. If you have access to it, you'll find that it gives an in-depth picture of the state of your recovery. Simply filling out the questionnaire may prompt some revelations about the balance between your training stress and recovery; scoring the form and graphing the answers will take you further.

With Tom Patrick, Cal Botterill, and Clare Wilson, Kellmann developed Recovery-Cue, a shorter questionnaire for athletes designed to be completed weekly.[4] Ideally, athletes would take the assessment at the same time each week, so that their answers are more consistent.

Recovery-Cue asks the following questions, with answers ranked numerically from 0 to 6; for your own use, you might choose a slightly different scale.

- How much effort was required to complete my workouts last week?
- How recovered did I feel before my workouts last week?
- How successful was I at rest and recovery activities this week?
- How well did I recover physically last week?
- How satisfied and relaxed was I as I fell asleep in the last week?
- How much fun did I have last week?
- How convinced was I that I could achieve my goals during performance last week?[5]

You need not be so detailed, however, to get an accurate sense of your recovery. Tracking qualitative data in metrics you design yourself can be effective, too. Here's how.

HOW TO TRACK RECOVERY YOURSELF
Your training log is an invaluable tool that shows trends over time. It can hold much more than numeric details on the miles you've covered or the wattage you've posted. Your log can become a journal, a record of your experiences day in and day out, a list of the small moments that make a life. Tracking indicators of your recovery will be invaluable in ensuring you reach peak performance in your key workouts and races. A few days' notes won't be of much use to you, but after you've accumulated data over a few weeks or months, you will see trends emerging.

Simply looking at your training log—miles and wattage and time—is not enough. You can be going through the same workouts but consistently under-recovering because of life stresses. Your sleep log might reveal a problem before your workout pacing does.

Figure 3.1 shows my athlete Donnie's log during the week he was tapering for a back-to-back mountain bike/duathlon race weekend. In a casual manner, he notes his sleep, nutrition, and the state of his legs. This is only one of the many ways in which you might track the quality of your recovery.

The means of tracking is up to you. If you prefer to work with a paper log, you might create a section in each day's listing where you rate these metrics. Or, periodically, take a pair of highlighters and work your way through your recent workout notes. Use one color—green, say—to highlight all the positive words you use, such as *strong, good, nailed it, excited*. Another color—safety orange, perhaps—can highlight any negative terms, such as *tired, sluggish, dead legs*, or *bad*. A glance at the color patterns will give you useful insights into trends.

If you are handy with Excel or other spreadsheets, you can create your own training log. You can program a formula so that your spreadsheet automatically computes your average metrics for the week, month, and year, such as the average hours slept per night, the rating you apply to stress, or your enjoyability score.

If you prefer an online log, you may be able to find metrics on hand that will help you measure the quality of your recovery. Training Peaks (trainingpeaks.com) has fields to track hours of sleep, weight, pulse, and percentage of body fat, along with dropdowns to input your stress level, sleep quality, fatigue, soreness, and "overall feeling." Training Peaks allows you to graph your daily metrics by plotting them against each other—that is, you can see your fatigue and sleep quality on the same graph.

Exactly how you track the factors that affect your recovery is less important than consistency in tracking.

WORKOUT	COMMENTS

Sunday, 10/10

Ride ~60 minutes, mostly easy, on a rolling course. Some pushing is okay on hills.
THEN, immediately off the bike, run 10 minutes or until your legs come around to feel like you're running, whichever comes first. You don't have to be fast, just try to stay upright with a quick turnover and think about making a smooth transition from bike to run.

Screwed up and didn't get my data started in time. Actually missed 25 minutes of some of my best riding in a year or two. Was taking it easy and still totally rocking it. Still did well for the next hour, and yes, that means I did more than you said, but was riding with Alan and really just having too much fun to stop. Tired, but not "too tired." Feel totally great, though. That's with exactly 8 hours sleep, which wasn't nearly enough. Gonna take a killer nap after some church and food, though. I mean, uh, "watch football." Yeah, that's the ticket.

Tuesday, 10/12

Back-and-forths. Warm up 15 minutes on the bike, winding up at a good transition place. Transition to the run, going 3 minutes. Back to the bike, ride out 3 minutes on an out-and back with the out effort easy and the back effort hard (i.e., under 3). Transition again and repeat, for a total of 3 runs, finishing with an easy bike.

The data is all here, but it's ugly to try to look at! Anyway, went just fine . . . nothing out of the ordinary. Might have felt a lot better if I had gotten up another 30 minutes earlier and had digested food in me, but no big deal.

Wednesday, 10/13

Warm up well, then 3 x just 3-minute race-pace efforts. Ride easily or even stop and catch your breath until you feel totally recovered between intervals. Easy ride as a cooldown.

Eh, having fun, rode fairly hard. Felt tired to start, but honestly I still felt really good. The "laps" were still kinda short, but I had trouble finding a loop closer to three minutes.

Thursday, 10/14

Warm up well, then run 6 x 30-second strides *down* a gentle hill. Jog easily to the starting point for recovery. Enjoy the feeling of quick turnover and speed with little effort—this is how we want the race to feel at its best moments. Cool down well, stretch, and get off your feet.

Boo to the weather for making me do this late in the day. Boo to myself for having blackened salmon and garlic fries for lunch. Boo to my knees for being mean to me. I dunno, they just don't feel good today. On the plus side, even feeling "not good" I still had a good average speed and great average cadence as I warmed up for the strides. I didn't feel like going all out, but I did just have a good cadence and good stride to move pretty fast. The hill wasn't very steep, but it was definitely all downhill. I also didn't jog back up . . . I walked about half then jogged the rest and turned immediately into the downhill.

Friday, 10/15

Stay off your feet as much as possible, and get a massage if you can. Take a few minutes today to sit quietly and review the way the races will play out: gear setup, warmups, transitions, terrain, how you will feel. If you're really antsy, practice your transitions, but avoid aerobic work today. Later in the day, enjoy these poses. Hold each for as long as you like, with special attention to resting with your legs up the wall.
*squatting on bolster
*reclining cobbler
*knees-down prone twist, belly to bolster
*bridge on block
*legs up the wall

Did it, loved it.

FIGURE 3.1
Donnie's log

Recovery Metrics to Note

Here are some ideas of metrics to note. Some may work for you, and others may not; what's important is consistent data collection so you can see trends emerge.

How's It Going?

In general, how is your training going? If the answer isn't an enthusiastic, honest "Great!" drill deeper. Are you in an intentional state of overreaching, working for a fitness breakthrough? How is that working out for you? Or are you simply pushing too hard? Are you having one or more failed workouts each week—workouts in which you can't make your target numbers, everything is off, or you blow up before you finish? Gordo Byrn, endurance coach and coauthor of *Going Long*, says that even though an occasional bad day is to be expected, "If you have more than one failed workout a week, you need to back off. One day a week is okay, but two is a sign."

Performance

Beyond the general perspective on how things are going, consider your performance in workouts. You should have target paces to hit for various distances in your workouts: Are you hitting the targets? Do they feel easy or tough to achieve? Comparing this effort to performance will give you a sense of how your training plan is working and whether you have sufficient recovery.

Body Quality

How do your muscles and lungs feel? Buoyant and clear? Heavy and congested? In his research, sport psychologist Jack Raglin uses a scale from 1 to 7 to describe the feeling of heaviness in limbs. "Swimmers feel like they're sinking in the water," he says; "runners have heavy legs. Come up with your own scale, and when you see a jump, that's when something is going on."

Mood

Mood fluctuations are a normal part of being human, but pay attention to your mood state. Big swings between good and bad moods should be noted, and any prolonged negative mood—be it tension, sadness, anger, depression, anxiety, or any other malaise—should be a red flag. When such moods persist, check your training and consider taking time off for recovery.

Sleeping

You can track both the amount of sleep you get—a quantifiable number—and the quality of your sleep. You might also note the extent of your dreaming. Do you awaken with memories of vivid dreams? If so, what are their common themes?

While it's normal to have a few nights where it's tough to fall asleep or to stay asleep, a regular pattern of subpar sleep is a warning sign. See chapter 8 for ways to improve the quality of your sleep.

External Stress

What kind of pressures are you currently under? Big deadline at work? In the midst of writing a dissertation? About to get married, start a new job, move cross-country, or undergo some other major life-changing event? These pressures will affect your training and your recovery, and they should be tracked.

Internal Stress

Internal stress is the pressure you put on yourself. It could be performance pressure, but it could also be pressure to succeed at work, to take care of a family member, to balance everything without showing strain. We all have internal stress. Sometimes simply making a note of it helps alleviate the problem. More about stress reduction appears in chapter 7.

Menstrual Cycle

Women should track their menstrual cycles, which can give insight into an athlete's state of recovery. A few missed periods or complete amenorrhea (complete absence of the period) are common indicators of overtraining. Female athletes can track their menstrual cycles in their training logs, noting the day the menses start, any abnormalities in flow or cramping, and duration. A change in any of these factors may be evidence of under-recovery. As trends emerge, the athlete or her coach might adjust training cycles so that rest weeks correspond with the week of the athlete's period, or the week just before. Once again, individuals must experiment to determine their individually appropriate combination of work and recovery.

Other Metrics

There may be other metrics you'd like to track. For example, one of my athletes who suffered from migraines appropriated the sleep metric in Training Peaks to track her migraine symptoms. If you have a cyclical work schedule—for example, a biweekly payroll day that keeps you very busy—it could be noted in your log, too.

Enjoyment

In *Run: The Mind-Body Method of Running by Feel*,[6] Matt Fitzgerald suggests tracking your enjoyment of each workout. Studies have shown that a lack of excitement for training can be one of the first signs of overtraining. Fitzgerald's system assigns a simple rating of 1 to 3 to your enjoyment of the workout, with 1 meaning it was on the whole unenjoyable, 2 meaning it was so-so, and 3 meaning it was an enjoyable experience. You can tally these points and divide them by the number of workouts to generate an enjoyability average for each week, month, and season. This is one example of how a simple metric gains power by being tracked over time. Single data points don't matter much; trends over time do.

PARTNER POWER

In addition to self-assessment, you can rely on those around you to let you know when you are pushing too much. If you have a coach, they should check in with you regularly to see how you're handling the workload. Ironman master coach Matt Dixon says he not only relies on his athletes' subjective self-assessments but also looks at the athletes themselves. Some details he notes are the vibrancy of an athlete's skin, attitude, and any moodiness. Even seemingly minor details, when added up, paint a picture of an athlete's recovery that an intuitive coach can evaluate. Stephen Seiler says, "One of the best ways for a coach to monitor athletes is just to observe their communication and personality. This is very low tech, and as a sport scientist, I wish the answer was some cool physiological measurement that only folks with PhDs could do, but that is not the case."

Many athletes never have face time with their coaches. If you're coached exclusively online, pay extra attention to communication with your coach. Don't hold back for fear of sounding like a whiner. Honest evaluation of your fatigue level is critically important to your training. Without full information on how your body is absorbing and adjusting to the prescribed workouts, a coach cannot design an intelligent progression toward your goals. At best, you'll fall shy of your potential if you are not fully recovered; at worst, you might be heading for injury or overtraining.

While well-known endurance sport coach Joe Friel's business is based online, he regularly monitors his athletes' training. He describes his process:

> I have [athletes] tell me how they feel in workouts. If they don't, then I send an e-mail asking about that. I talk with them once a week to hear how enthusiastic, tired, stressed, happy, sad, or excited they are. I also teach them what to look for and always encourage them in the training plan to cut back on a given workout if they don't feel like working hard or long. When they do reduce the workload, I praise them for being smart enough to make a good decision. But they never have permission to unilaterally make the workout harder.

Coach Mike Ricci finds that online work can make the coach's assessment tougher. "One of the best things about coaching athletes in person is being able to see them," he says. "Seeing how their body language is, how their form is, energy level, and even just to look into their eyes to gauge the state of fatigue."

If you don't meet with a coach in person or speak with one regularly, ask your friends and family members to keep an eye on you. They can let you know if they notice a shift in your appearance, mood, or mental acuity. Byrn calls this a "reality check" from someone who knows you well—a wife, husband, boyfriend, girlfriend, training buddy, or friend. "It may be apparent to those people before it is to the athlete," he says.

ADJUSTING TRAINING BASED ON THESE MEASUREMENTS

If you discern that you are not recovering as planned, back off. It could mean a number of different things. Sometimes, taking a few days or a week of complete rest is the best plan. That means no workouts at all; in fact, it may even be best to take a complete time-out from even thinking about training. (Naturally, this is easier said than done.)

Other times, you might follow the same cycle of your workouts—keeping swim/bike days as swim/bike days, for example—but completely eliminate intensity. Thus your body and mind have the routine of enjoying your daily activity, but without any additional stress. Leave out your main sets and intervals; the entire workout should be done at the same easy intensity you use for warm-up and cooldown.

After a week of lighter workouts or no workouts, reassess your metrics. Has your sleep improved? Your mood? Did you enjoy these lighter workouts? Depending on your answers, another few days or another week of intensity-free workouts might be in order. If you feel ready to resume harder work, slide back into it gently, keeping a close eye on your mood and your other metrics to determine whether you are sufficiently recovered or need a little longer.

QUICK TIPS

- Tracking your mood, sleep quality, and other metrics gives you insight into the state of your recovery.

- A coach, spouse, or close friend will have valuable insight into how well you are handling your training load. Listen.

- If you feel things coming off the rails, adjust your training for a few days and reassess.

4

Quantitative Measurements of Recovery

As we saw in chapter 3, much of recovery is qualitative and can't easily be measured, and qualitative predictors often work before a problem in recovery can be quantified. But there are some ways to quantify recovery, as we examine in this chapter. Like any training technology, these are tools to help you get to know your body and its needs. The tools give you a window of insight, but you must ultimately make a decision by weighing both quantitative and qualitative input.

Many of these tools measure recovery indirectly, by quantifying its absence. For example, a rise in resting heart rate (RHR) or a high Training Stress Score in WKO5, described later in the chapter, indicates stress on the body rather than recovery. Many of these tests suggest over-reaching or the onset of overtraining. Focusing on adequate recovery using the tools and techniques outlined in part II may eventually help you avoid the need for such testing entirely.

The home testing tools described here grow progressively more complicated, and some require comfort with math and technology. If they confuse you, they may not be right for you. You will do just fine with a qualitative impression of your recovery and an emphasis on training smart, increasing sleep, reducing stress, and eating well. If you'd like to try some of the more complicated methods, you'll probably find they confirm what you already suspected about the state of your recovery. In fact, that is how they are best deployed: as a confirmation of what you already know and plan to do next, not as a backseat driver goading you to make poor choices based on single data points.

LABORATORY TESTS

One way athletes can quantify their recovery is to undergo periodic blood lactate testing. Most sports performance laboratories, many fitness centers, and some coaches offer it. Such testing is useful for establishing training zones based on pace or heart rate, so that athletes can use these parameters in workouts targeting specific energy systems. But blood lactate can also indicate the onset of overtraining. A 1993 study showed that when an athlete begins to overreach, a blood lactate test will show lower levels of lactate concentration compared to ratings of perceived exertion.[1] That is, work begins to feel more taxing than it measures, physiologically.

When overtraining syndrome is suspected, a doctor may order more sophisticated tests, including an assessment of mitochondria function and various hormonal tests to check levels of cortisol and human growth hormone as well as the state of the adrenal glands. These tests require direct medical supervision and do not measure day-to-day recovery. Instead, they are deployed in cases of severe under-recovery.

Athletes at the U.S. Olympic Training Centers and other elite facilities have the luxury of having blood work done to assess their adaptation. Coaches can look for various indicators, such as iron levels, that show whether an athlete is recovering from training stresses. But such testing is out of the reach of most athletes. Luckily, the average athlete can quantify recovery through various home tests.

HOME TESTS WITH SIMPLE DEVICES

Each of these home tests is fairly straightforward, but they grow progressively more detailed. Most important for your quantification of recovery is consistent measurement, regardless of the test you are using. No single data point means much; having many data points that you can read in context can be very powerful. Trends over time matter more than any single piece of information.

Resting Heart Rate

One simple test to measure recovery is by tracking your RHR. This can be done every morning before rising, provided that conditions are the same. Such a test presumes that you have awoken without a harsh alarm sound, which could cause a stress reaction and skew the results. The heart rate can be measured with a manual count, with a finger-clamp pulse reader (sold as pulse oximeters at medical-supply stores), with a smartwatch or ring, or with a heart-rate monitor. In the latter case, rest a few minutes after donning the monitor strap so your heart rate can return to stasis. Alternatively, at some established point in the day well separated from exercise, lie down for a few minutes, then measure your resting heart rate.

Note this number in your training log. After tracking your heart rate for a week or more, an average resting heart rate should become apparent. If a day's measurement is 5 to 10 beats higher than usual, it could be a sign of elevated stress, either through training or because of an impending infection; more rest or an easy day of workouts is in order. Some coaches recommend switching to an easy workout with a 5-beat spike in RHR, and dropping the workout entirely with a 10-beat spike. Depending on your personal resting heart rate, however, these numbers can carry more or less meaning. If you have a resting heart rate of 35, for example, 5 beats is a more significant change than if your resting heart rate is 70. Time will give you a sense of what change in resting heart rate is acceptable. Remember that your heart rate will be affected by a number of factors, from the state of your training and recovery to your mood, the quality and duration of your sleep, the strength of your immune system, and your nutritional status. While these latter factors have an effect on your recovery, they may be related to other things happening in your life, so you must look at resting heart rate as one part of a bigger picture.

Orthostatic Heart Rate Test

The orthostatic (standing upright) heart rate test developed by Finnish exercise physiologist Heikki Rusko compares the resting heart rate with the heart rate after a shift in position and the subsequent ambient heart rate standing. To perform the test, lie down while wearing your heart rate monitor, whether it's a watch, strap, ring, finger clamp, or other wearable. After a few minutes of rest, you'll see your heart rate stabilize. Time 2 minutes here as you recline, then stand up and note your heart rate at 15 seconds, 90 seconds, and 120 seconds after standing. If your monitor gives an average heart rate for the period between 90 and 120 seconds after standing, all the better. Note these numbers in your log.

Figure 4.1 illustrates the curve of your heart rate after you make the switch to standing. You will see that your heart rate spikes about 15 seconds after you make the shift from reclining to standing and then levels off. Rusko found that athletes on the verge of overtraining exhibit a higher average heart rate than normal in the period between 90 and 120 seconds after standing, which is evidence of strain on the sympathetic

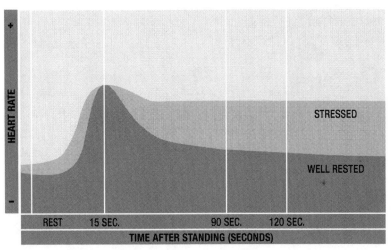

FIGURE 4.1
Curve of heart rate

nervous system. This indicates that a stress load has been added to the body beyond its ability to adapt. As with resting heart rate, this test is most effective when performed regularly over time. You might want to include this test daily or weekly. Aim to create the same circumstances each time: Measure at the same time of day and on the same day of each training microcycle.

TRACKING DEVICES AND WEARABLES

Many athletes now train with GPS smartwatches, fitness trackers, or other wearables like rings that measure heart rate, heart rate variability, temperature, SpO2, and more. This field changes rapidly. Sian Allen, PhD, an expert in wearable technology, explains that the hardware is far ahead of the software right now. In the years to come, she expects software to evolve to become "more akin to a coach in your pocket that actually can provide individualized recommendations and insight into your data, beyond the generic commentary that exists right now."

As researcher Robert Furberg, who currently works in tracking devices for the Divers' Awareness Network, puts it, "These devices make collecting a lot of data very easy, collecting good data very hard, and collecting very good data that's both meaningful and actionable very, very hard. There's so much individual variation that it's no surprise people are like, 'Weird, my watch says . . .' It's a vicious cycle, because there's a massive market that keeps growing and growing and most of the work that remains to be done is on the back end. You have all this data, so what?"

Here's what: Don't fixate on any particular data point lest you miss the forest for the trees. Instead, look for trends over time. Allen says, "The biggest mistake I see across the board is not understanding or questioning where there's error of measurement in a device or a metric, and therefore risking attributing value to noise instead of signal. You have to understand the error of measurement you're dealing with to understand what a meaningful change in a metric is, and then you need to interpret it with the right context in order to be able to act upon it appropriately." These errors in measurement can range from software glitches to LEDs' poor performance in measuring data from darker skin tones, so you will do well to use your data as only one part of a full-spectrum assessment that includes plenty of qualitative information about how you feel and how you are performing.

Marco Altini, PhD, who has a background in data science, computer science engineering, and sports science, agrees. He says that while data collection is now easy, data interpretation "is still often misguided or very naïve—for example, using a simple 'higher is better' approach—or providing the data without the required context, like a normal range individual to the athlete." He emphasizes how important it is to collect several weeks' worth of data to define an individually normal range. Only then can we be "able to determine which day-to-day changes are meaningful (e.g., outside of the normal range) and which changes are just part of day-to-day variability in these metrics. When we are able to do so, then we can use the data effectively."

Heart Rate Variability

Heart rate variability (HRV) refers to the difference in the time between individual heartbeats. When your heart is beating at 60 beats per minute, the time between individual beats isn't necessarily one second. Rather, the space between beats can change from 0.89 seconds to 1.23 seconds and so on. This variability is a positive thing: It shows that the parasympathetic nervous system is in control and that the body is under a relatively light load of stress. When the beats come more regularly and with less variability, the system is under stress. In fact, low heart rate variability is often a precursor to a cardiac event such as a heart attack. But this stress can also come from exercise, so HRV is not relevant during exercise. Instead, it's measured at rest, to determine how ready the heart is to adjust to the body's needs moment to moment.

Heart rate variability can thus be a good indicator of recovery. The greater the variability, the more recovered the athlete. Many smartwatches, fitness trackers, and heart rate monitors now give a heart rate variability measurement—though it is actually, as researcher Robert Furberg points out, a pulse rate variability measurement, because of the limitations of the technology. (For real HRV measurements, you'd use an ECG machine to measure the electrical impulses in your heart.) Altini developed and validated a way to measure HRV using a smartphone camera. It's built in to his app, HRV4Training, which combines subjective measurements to give users a sense of their readiness to train. You place your finger over the camera lens for a short time and receive an HRV measurement.

Know, however, that like resting heart rate, heart rate variability can change for a number of reasons, and the state of your recovery is only one of them. Altini explains, "Using the data effectively typically means being able to detect when we have a negative response (e.g., a suppressed HRV, below an athlete's normal range), and aiming for stability, as a stable HRV highlights an ideal response. This is true even when training hard, and is maybe one of the most poorly understood aspects: a stable HRV does not represent a lack of stress but highlights a great ability of the system to respond and renormalize quickly. On the other hand, an unstable HRV or low HRV the day after training highlights a mismatch between the stimulus and the athlete's fitness—time to rethink the training plan—or the presence of non-training-related stressors." Chapter 7, on stress reduction, will help you with ways to identify and manage your life stresses.

Excess Postexercise Oxygen Consumption

Excess postexercise oxygen consumption (EPOC) occurs in the period immediately after exercise, when the body takes in extra oxygen—in excess of that used by the metabolism at rest—to compensate for the effect of the exercise and to bring the system back into homeostasis. As such, the amount of EPOC predicts the amount of stress that a workout has placed on the body. EPOC can be measured in a lab by examining an athlete's gaseous intake and output with a mask, but that is obviously inconvenient for daily use. Many training watches now estimate the amount of EPOC associated with a given workout and therefore suggest the amount of recovery that should be taken afterward. Depending on the brand and model, the watches may display this in various ways. Any athlete using one of these monitors should compare the data from the monitor to their own sense of perceived exertion. When the monitor's take on your training load in a workout is high and in line with perceived exertion, the stress from the workout indicates that attention should be paid to recovery. A disconnect between your monitor's load assessment and your perceived exertion, in which the reported load is low but exertion feels high, can indicate a need for more recovery before performing another intense workout. A correlated low monitored load and low perceived exertion suggest that the athlete should increase intensity to encourage positive adaptation. But take every number as what it is: simply one data point. Trust your brain and your gut over your watch, and trends across time over single instances.

Foster's Modified Rating of Perceived Exertion

If you're game for assessing your own training load, Carl Foster, an exercise physiologist emeritus at the University of Wisconsin–La Crosse, developed a method to quantify training load based on the Rating of Perceived Exertion scale created by Gunnar Borg. While the Borg scale rates the effort one perceives to be giving at the moment on a scale from 6 to 20 (numbers selected to correspond roughly to heart rates of 60 and 200), Foster's scale applies that same metric to the *entire* workout, using a scale modified to go from 0 to 10.

To use the system, assign a number from 0 to 10 to rate the intensity of your workout, with 0 being no effort and 10 a maximal effort. (Foster advises waiting about 30 minutes before rating your workout.) Then multiply that number by the number of minutes the workout lasted. For example, a two-hour-long run that felt like a 3, a pretty moderate effort, would rate 360 training load units for the session (120 × 3). A short, hard bike ride with several all-out efforts might last 45 minutes but rate a 9, yielding 405 units (45 × 9). You can even quantify nonaerobic workouts in the same way. A weightlifting session might last 50 minutes with an intensity of 6: 50 × 6 = 300; a yoga workshop might be 180 minutes with an intensity of 4: 180 × 4 = 720.

These calculations are easy to make, and they involve your own perception of how hard the workout was, thus taking into account the other stressors you're under—something your watch or other wearable monitor may not be able to capture. Foster says that even though his approach is not as exact as E. W. Banister's training impulse system (TRIMP), described later in the chapter, it's simpler: "If you missed a night's sleep last night because your kids weren't sleeping, that integrates the other things going on in your life. If you didn't get a good meal and your legs are glycogen depleted, it's going to show up."

Once you've accumulated data over several days, some simple analysis can give you fascinating insights by looking at the monotony of your training—whether or not there is variety in your training load. Training monotony is correlated with overtraining, and carrying a load above the average amount of strain the athlete is accustomed to often leads to illness. Monitoring the variation across the week can allow an athlete to carry a higher load of strain without becoming ill or overtrained, as "multiple 'easy' days within each week may allow a given training load to be accomplished with comparatively fewer negative outcomes."[2] Foster explains that the training load of 4,000 units per week, which is about what many elites are carrying—four hard days per week, interspersed with two easy days and an off day—greatly reduces training strain compared to six hard days and one off day.

You can calculate the standard deviation (the nearness to the mean) of your daily training load using an online calculator (or longhand, if you're statistically minded). To figure the monotony of your training load, divide the daily average by the standard deviation. To determine your weekly load, multiply the daily average by seven. (Log a zero for a full rest day with no workouts, as that will affect your standard deviation.) Finally, to calculate your strain, multiply your weekly load by the monotony of the week. Tracking this number across time will demonstrate to you your personal threshold for strain, and when you cross it, you'll be in the red zone, starting to exhibit less recovery and in danger of overtraining.

While this sounds complicated, if you're handy with a spreadsheet, you can create an easy way to track your load, monotony, and training strain. (I've done just that for you: find the downloadable file at sage rountree.com/recovery.) Tables 4.1 and 4.2 show two training weeks. In table 4.1, I've tallied the training load of a week I logged while training to run the New York Marathon. In table 4.2, I've outlined a highly monotonous (and hard!) training week for comparison's sake. While this is a hypothetical week, it's representative of many athletes' reality. You'll see that the total load between the two is virtually identical—my week rated 2,065, while the other week rated 2,080. But notice the difference in the standard deviation of the daily load, which has a huge effect on the monotony of the weeks. My week had a monotony number of 1.5, while the run-hard-every-day week rated more than

Table 4.1. Sample training load for one week

DAY	WORKOUT	DURATION IN MINUTES	RATING OF PERCEIVED EXERTION (RPE)	LOAD (DURATION X RPE)
Monday	Run with pickups	40	5	200
	Swim	30	3	90
	Yoga	60	2	120
Tuesday	Cycling moderate	50	3	150
	Run easy	30	3	90
Wednesday	Run with intervals	45	7	315
	Swim	40	2	80
	Yoga	60	2	120
Thursday	Cycling easy	50	2	100
Friday	Run easy	40	2	80
Saturday	Run long with fast finish	120	6	720
Sunday	Off	0	0	0
Daily load				2,065
Daily average load (total load ÷ 7)				295
Standard deviation of daily load				188
Monotony (daily average load ÷ standard deviation)				1.5
Strain (total load × monotony)				3,097

Table 4.2. Sample hard training load for one week

DAY	WORKOUT	DURATION IN MINUTES	RATING OF PERCEIVED EXERTION (RPE)	LOAD (DURATION X RPE)
Monday	Run	60	5	300
Tuesday	Run	60	5	300
Wednesday	Run	60	5	300
Thursday	Run	60	5	300
Friday	Run	60	5	300
Saturday	Run	70	4	280
Sunday	Run	60	5	300
Total load				2,080
Daily average load (total load ÷ 7)				297
Standard deviation of daily load				7.0
Monotony (daily average load ÷ standard deviation)				42.4
Strain (total load × monotony)				88,192

28 times higher, at 42.4. And while I carried a training strain of 3,097, our poor imaginary runner's strain rates 88,192. The implication is obvious: It is much more stressful to go hard each day than to alternate hard and easy workouts.

SOFTWARE FOR MEASURING RECOVERY

TRIMP

By quantifying the training load, athletes can track the amount of stress put on their bodies and match their recovery to meet the workload. One way to do so is kinesiologist E. W. Banister's training impulse (TRIMP) system, which measures training dosage as duration times delta heart rate ratio, where the delta heart rate ratio equals the average heart rate during exercise, minus RHR, divided by the athlete's maximum heart rate, minus RHR (equation 4.1):

$$\mathit{delta\ HR} = \frac{\mathit{av.\ HR\ during\ exercise - RHR}}{\mathit{max.\ HR - RHR}}$$

TRIMP can then be tracked in a spreadsheet. You'll find one you can download at sagerountree.com/recovery.

WKO

Assessment of training load (and thus the need for recovery) is robustly covered by WKO, a proprietary software application that is linked to the Training Peaks website. Currently on version WKO5, the software tracks the effect of training metrics on the performance of endurance athletes and allows athletes and their coaches to manipulate training based on a quantifiable amount of stress put on the body. Based on input from power- and pace-measuring devices such as power meters and speed-and-distance watches, WKO software assigns a few numeric values to each workout, including Intensity Factor (IF) and Training Stress Score (TSS). It then combines these numbers with data over time to measure an athlete's Chronic Training Load (CTL) and Acute Training Load (ATL)—or, as Training Peaks says, an athlete's fitness and freshness.

To use the training stress measurements, an athlete needs access to technology and energy for field testing, as well as a power meter for bike workouts and a pace-sensing watch (such as a GPS-enabled watch) for running. Alternatively, athletes can estimate the effect of a given workout and enter its stress manually. For uploaded data, Dr. Andrew Coggan's Training Stress Score (TSS) weights workouts' effect on the body, given the athlete's functional threshold power—the best average amount of wattage generated in one hour's cycling. A running Training Stress Score (rTSS), based on functional threshold pace—the maximum sustainable pace for an hour's run—serves the same purpose. These numbers then inform the CTL and ATL. When CTL is high and ATL is low, the athlete is probably feeling fresh and recovered. When ATL is high in relationship to CTL (whether CTL is itself a high or a low number), an athlete's body is in need of recovery for peak performance.

The relationship between chronic and acute fatigue—between CTL and ATL—is the Training Stress Balance (TSB). Physiologist Stephen McGregor, who helped develop analytical tools for WKO+, says, "The TSB value is the most important thing in regards to looking at your recovery. Especially for a self-coached user, that's the real value. It's difficult for an individual to maintain objectivity. They're too close to their training; they're too invested. The quantitative approach in WKO+ allows people to get an objective, broader perspective."

Figure 4.2, generated in WKO+, shows the performance management chart for my athlete Stacey, an elite age-group triathlete. At the end of June, she did a heavy cycling-intensive block, and then we pulled her training back to prep for a B-priority race on July 10. She performed wonderfully at the race, especially on the bike—and you can see from the TSB line spiking higher that she was feeling pretty fresh coming in to the race.

The various commercial software options each use slightly different formulas and slightly different interfaces. If you are interested in using

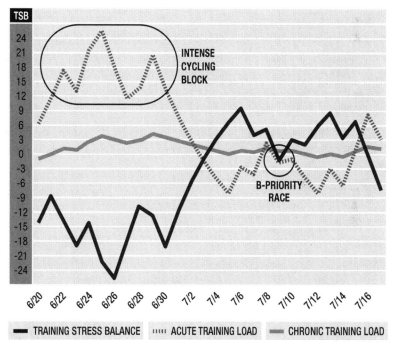

FIGURE 4.2
Performance management chart

Note: Training stress balance is low as the acute training load is high; they swap positions as an athlete enters a lighter training block in preparation for a race.

them to track your training load, you'll need to try each out and make a choice based on your technical abilities, computer, and needs. The more data you can accrue in these applications, the more powerful the application becomes. You will be able to see trends: What level of acute training load can you maintain? What is too much? How much time do you need for recovery after workouts of various intensities? Use the technology to help you hone your awareness of your own body, rather than fixating on any single data point to dictate what you do.

Marco Altini says, "We can get better at understanding our body and using subjective feel for guidance by using data. Our awareness will improve as we start paying more attention and use, for example, heart rate variability as an objective marker of physiological stress." These quantitative tools help by confirming our innate impressions. Sian Allen agrees. Before you look at your numbers, she suggests, "take a few minutes to check in with yourself. If you had to give yourself a score for how recovered you feel, what would it be? Then open your app and see how close you are and reflect on where the differences or similarities are. This process of 'interoceptive journaling' is intended to help athletes get closer to being in tune with their own bodies, such that the data can help calibrate their own inner sense of recovery. I think the best tech helps promote self-reliance and human growth, rather than just dependence!"

LOGGING

For any of these home tests to be effective, you'll need to keep careful track of your metrics. This can happen on paper, in a spreadsheet on your computer, or in an online log or an app. If you track your resting heart rate, orthostatic heart rate, or heart rate variability, each of these numbers should be noted. A few words describing what other stressors are at play that day will help you observe trends as they emerge (see chapter 3). Over weeks, months, and years of logging, you'll generate a powerful database for insight into your body and its performance.

QUICK TIPS

- The best quantitative measurements are those you will use consistently, so you can track data over time.

- You can get sophisticated with your measurements, but they will likely ultimately reflect your intuition about the state of your recovery.

5

Recovery from Injury and Illness

This book focuses on recovery for healthy and uninjured people between workouts. But sometimes healthy and uninjured people take ill or become injured. The recovery process from illness and injury is unique to the individual and should be managed between the individual athlete and his or her health care practitioners, including physical therapists in the event of injury.

To complement your work with your own support team, however, here are some general guidelines.

PREVENTION

Rule one: Prevent illness and injury before they start. This is, of course, easier said than done, even in a world where masking has been normalized. It involves paying close attention to your body and hitting the pause button on your training as soon as you notice something a little out of the ordinary: a tickle in your throat, a niggle in your knee. Sometimes, a day or two of lighter or no training will boost your recovery and ward off illness or injury. If you've rested a day or two but do not improve or your symptoms worsen with training, head to the clinic.

Hal Rosenberg, a member of the USA Triathlon medical staff, suggests using this rule of thumb when something starts to hurt: Ask yourself if the symptom is affecting your biomechanics. If you find yourself moving in different patterns to avoid pain, you should cease the activity. Don't wait until things worsen before consulting with a health care provider. Rosenberg explains:

> A lot of the problems we see in the sports medicine world are people with injuries they think they can train through, but it worsens and there are compensation injuries. The sooner people address these problems, the more successful they can become at resolving them. Some athletes seek care at the last minute before an A-race with a problem that's been going on for a while. Best-case scenario, we patch them up so they can simply complete the race. If they'd addressed it at the onset, we could have gotten them healed so they can race at their potential.

Be honest with yourself when you feel something is amiss. Having a coach or a loved one give you an honest assessment is very helpful. If you suspect something is wrong but don't have an advocate arguing for you to rest and take the time to heal, it's very easy to shrug off the pain or ache and train anyway. This can be the start of a chain of trouble, from a change in your stride or stroke or technique to further strain on your immune system. The clichés are right: Nip it in the bud. A stitch in time saves nine. Better safe than sorry.

DISTINGUISHING INJURY FROM SORENESS

As training necessarily carries with it some strain on your system to induce supercompensation, it's normal to experience some pain and soreness, especially during periods of heavy training load. The trick is finding ways to distinguish between normal soreness and signs of an impending injury.

If you feel soreness or tenderness in the center of your muscles, and you feel it on both sides of your body, it's likely normal. If you feel pain localized toward a joint (in the tendons or in the ligaments of the joint itself) or only on one side of your body, beware. If the pain comes on after a workout with new movements or one that is more intense or longer than usual, keep an eye on it. It should improve in a day or two.

Table 5.1.   Soreness as a warning sign

NORMAL SORENESS	WARNING SIGN
On both sides of the body	On one side of the body
Felt in the center of a muscle	Felt toward a joint
Appears after a change in workout intensity, duration, or modality	Appears daily
Improves after warm-up	Worsens during workout
Improves daily	Worsens or remains daily
Doesn't affect your form	Affects your form
Generalized	Localized

If the pain continues to worsen or you feel it during exercise, especially if it affects your form, stop and have it evaluated. Table 5.1 lists the difference between normal soreness and warning signs you should keep your eye on.

RECOVERY FROM INJURY AND ILLNESS

If you find yourself with an injury or illness that interferes with your training, be very careful about your return to workouts. A common psychological trap is to worry about your perceived loss of fitness. (While high-end speed will fade after a week or two of disuse, your muscular and aerobic endurance will still be present after a few weeks or even a month off.) Often, what seems like a loss of fitness is the effect of the illness—you can easily still be dehydrated from a stomach bug or have problems breathing after a respiratory infection. You need to be able to train pain and symptom free to make the quickest rebound. That might mean bailing on workouts, resting, and trying again in a day or two, and this cycle may be repeated many times.

Your recovery will differ, depending on what sidetracked you. A 24-hour bout of vomiting will leave you weak and knock you out of training, but you'll probably be able to step back in to your training plan after a day or two of lighter workouts. Recovery from the flu might mean two weeks of missed workouts. Returning from a cracked rib might take a month or more, and a pelvic stress fracture or COVID-19 can mean months of rehabilitation. Resist the urge to return too soon, which may only exacerbate the problem, taking you right back to square one or, even worse, setting you back further. Better to be patient than to remain injured because of a hasty return.

Returning to low-impact sports such as swimming and cycling can happen once you are symptom free. Take it easy and slowly, with short and light workouts, increasing intensity after a few days. Carefully and honestly assess your progress and back off if you get warning signs from the site of injury or the symptoms of illness return.

Returning to a running program requires special care because running is a high-impact activity; returning to contact sports after an injury will be even trickier. Happily, athletes in contact sports usually work with an athletic trainer and coaches who can assess their progress and ease them back on to the field. Self- or remotely coached endurance athletes who run will need to be very disciplined in their return. Consult with a physical therapist and your health care team to find the best strategy for you.

Recovery from an Overuse Injury

Recovery from an overuse injury will depend on what was hurt. Some soft-tissue irritation can be alleviated pretty quickly, while a stress fracture will take weeks or months to heal. Most important in your recovery from an overuse injury will be understanding the cause of the problem. All overuse injuries happen because of an imbalance— usually, an imbalance in your body. A biomechanist or a physical therapist skilled in working with athletes can help you address the root problem, usually through strengthening and flexibility exercises. Technique drills can then reinforce the correct movement pattern. Some of this work can be done while you are recovering; it will continue once you resume training.

Some overuse injuries are caused by using the wrong equipment: swim paddles that send too much force to your shoulders; a bike fit that has your saddle too high, too low, too far forward, or too far back; or running shoes that are too old or not suitable for your gait. These problems can usually be corrected sooner, and avoiding them is easy if you periodically check in with experts who know how to assess bike fit or running shoes.

Recovery from an Acute Injury

Acute injuries usually result from a fall or a crash. The time needed for proper healing and recovery depends on what is banged up and the level of inflammation and pain you're experiencing. Sometimes, cross-training is a good way to maintain your aerobic fitness while you heal. A runner with a sprained ankle might be comfortable riding a bike; a cyclist with a broken collarbone might be okay riding the trainer; a swimmer with a broken wrist might enjoy hiking.

Recovery from Illness

Your recovery from illness depends on the severity and duration of the illness and on what systems it affected. You can train lightly with symptoms from the neck up—a sore throat, a stuffy nose, a headache—but should not train with symptoms that affect areas below the neck. That includes a cough, a fever, and gastrointestinal trouble. When you have these whole-body symptoms, you need to let them abate before you consider training, and if training makes things worse, resting is preferable. Your body will give you the cues you need about whether to go or stop. Listen to your body instead of your head, which may try to rush you back to training too soon.

Recovery from COVID-19

Since the onset of the COVID-19 pandemic, medical professionals and coaches have had to design new approaches for return to training after an infection with SARS-COV-2. While return-to-training guidelines continue to evolve, a quick internet search will point you toward the most recent thinking.[1]

If your symptoms persist longer than you expect, or if your fatigue level seems high after activity, check in with your health care team, and ideally also with a practitioner who has experience with helping other COVID-19 patients in a graduated return to exercise.

QUICK TIPS

- Pay attention to warning signs from your body. Dropping a few workouts to rest at the first sign of injury or illness is more productive than missing weeks down the road when you are seriously hurt or sick.

- Work with your health care team to address the root problem that led to an overuse injury.

- Don't train through symptoms of illness that appear below the neck—congestion in the lungs, fever, or gastrointestinal distress.

- Make a slow, methodical return to training after time off and reduce your training if your symptoms recur.

Part II

RECOVERY TECHNIQUES

6

Active Recovery

Time: little to moderate

Cost: free

Accessibility: good

Confidence: good

Contraindications: extreme soreness that affects movement

WHAT CONSTITUTES ACTIVE RECOVERY

Active recovery is exercise at a low intensity. It has many rightful places: within a workout (for example, jogging easily between intervals), immediately after a workout (the cooldown), and as a stand-alone training session. Some even use the phrase "active recovery" to refer to the off-season. Studies have demonstrated its benefit in all these contexts.

Our concern here is not with active recovery between bouts of exercise such as intervals on the track or events in a swim meet, where it's proven to help with short-term recovery.[1] Rather, we're interested in the benefits of the cooldown and of scheduled easy training sessions.

The Cooldown

A 2000 study showed that an easy cooldown performed after running at moderate intensity for two sets of an hour each, or high intensity for two half-hour sets, helped prevent the fall of white blood cell count that happens in the first 15 minutes after exercise.[2] The implication here is that the cooldown helps your systems gently return to normal and reduces stress on your immune system. Think of the cooldown as you would turning off your computer by choosing "shut down" from your computer's main menu, rather than simply yanking the power-cord plug from the socket. As the computer shuts down in stages, it cleans itself up—putting files where they belong, closing applications one by one. Your body does the same during cooldown. It clears lactic acid pretty quickly—faster with cooldown than without—and helps all the systems return to homeostasis.[3] Your body temperature comes back to normal more smoothly, your central nervous system calms down, and you prepare for your recovery. Simply stopping is a greater shock to your system.

Follow your cooldown with some gentle static stretching, holding each stretch for 30 seconds or five slow breaths. Taking advantage of your warmer muscles, you can use this opportunity to improve your range of motion. (Static stretching isn't advised *before* a workout, when dynamic, movement-based stretching is better, but it still has its place.) For short postworkout routines appropriate for athletes, please see my book *Everyday Yoga*.

Easy Training Sessions

Easy, stand-alone active recovery workouts elevate the heart rate just enough to increase blood flow to recovering muscles, and they must be light enough so that they do not tax the muscular and cardiovascular systems they are intended to help.

Scheduled easy sessions should consist of light-intensity workouts and can involve your primary sport or a different, lower-impact modality. (See below for some ideas.) The intensity must be quite light. If you train with heart rate using the five-zone system outlined in Joe Friel's *Training Bible* books, active recovery would be in zone 1—that is, no higher than 55 percent of your maximum heart rate. Friel refers to his easy rides as "taking a walk on the bike." You should be able to speak a monologue during your active recovery sessions—the effort should be completely conversational. I sometimes tell my athletes that they may want to shower afterward, but they shouldn't need to wash their hair. The effort, then, is just enough to break a sweat. The session shouldn't last much longer than a half hour. Beyond about 40 minutes, you're moving into an easy endurance workout rather than an active recovery session.

Space your recovery workouts to come between days of hard training, or, if you do multiple workouts in a day, about 12 hours after a hard workout and 12 before your next one. Your individual need for recovery and your ability to handle harder training will dictate how often you need active recovery sessions. They may follow one of the patterns laid out in chapter 1, or you might find that a different sequence works for you. What's important is including them and keeping your training from drifting into moderate-hard intensity every day.

The cyclicality of hard alternating with easy plays out not only in the day and the week but also across training cycles and even across years. Think of Olympians who take an easy year or two in their quadrennial cycles. Check that there is variety across your training at every level, from the cooldown after a hard workout to the easier year after a particularly tough season. Active recovery, both in easy workouts and in easy days, introduces variability to training. Remember Carl Foster's finding, outlined in chapter 4, that athletes can adapt better to a greater overall training stress when it is variable instead of monotonous. Make the easy days really easy so that the hard days can be truly hard. If you can rein in your effort on your easy days, you'll have room to push a little faster or a little longer on your hard days, yielding a much bigger fitness reward than simply muddling through with easy days that are too hard and hard days that therefore become too slow or short. Foster remembers, "[legendary running coach] Jack Daniels was my professor in school. He is famous for apparently undertraining his athletes, but they all seem to get good results." Foster recalls physiologist Stephen Seiler's quote: "If you don't rest on the easy days, you won't be able to train hard enough on the hard days to improve." Complete rest would beat blowing a planned easy run or spin by getting sucked into a pace that's faster than intended.

Of course, this is easier said than done, given the psychology of athletes, especially in group situations. Foster reviewed various coaches' plans, comparing them to how hard the athletes actually trained. While the plans had an appropriate balance of work and rest, hard days and easy days, the athletes had trouble following the plan as written. "Most coaches are very smart people," Foster said. "They occupy the same niche as physicians: they diagnose problems and create a prescription to fix them. Most serious coaches are serious people. [Looking at] the results, on the days the coaches wanted to go easy, the athletes every time went harder. So when the coaches wanted to go hard, the athletes couldn't." Foster's review consistently shows that athletes don't take the easy days that allow them to go hard when they need to.

If you know you are susceptible to such racing in practice, excuse yourself from the group and instead do your own thing. Or spend this time with a slower friend—the one who's always apologizing for holding you back. Better still, run or ride with a child, provided it's a slow-moving child!

Don't discount the power of a day completely off or filled only with some very light walking, especially if you find it hard to go easy. How much recovery you need will be specific to you, depending on your age, history with the sport, workouts, and more. Weekend warriors will need more; professional athletes may need less, and it might involve active rest more than passive rest. Physiologist Stephen Seiler says,

It seems that the more an athlete trains, the less complete rest they need. When an athlete has a hormonal and biological rhythm built around very frequent training, complete rest days actually seem to disturb that rhythm in the short term. That is, the workout after a complete rest day may feel rotten for an athlete training 13 sessions a week. That does not mean that complete rest days are not useful for elite athletes, but it does mean that they are unlikely to actually use complete rest prior to competition, surprisingly enough. On the other hand, a recreational athlete who puts in a hard weekend of training that is clearly over their normal physical stress load will need that complete rest day on Monday.

Coach Matt Dixon, CEO and founder of Purple Patch Fitness, has a protocol for his athletes incorporating easy sessions as well as programmed rest. He explains, "You can actually leverage training to be a decompression tool to the other stresses in life." In a plan, he says, "We have multiple sessions each week where I'm willing to forgo a little bit of specificity and a little bit of focus, if the athlete can go for an easy run and do whatever they'd like to do. For me, that would be listening to a podcast or an audio book. I'm still getting general cardiovascular conditioning and health benefits from moving blood around, and I'm getting some tissue resilience. But I'm actually getting emotional recovery. Because we have so many competing demands for our attention." For active recovery, Dixon says, "frequent is okay; long is bad."

Coach Peter Magill agrees. He describes an active recovery session:

Not longer than 40 minutes, not shorter than 20 minutes, done at an effort level lighter than normal. Still with the normal stride—not too slow—but a little bit easier. We get circulation going, lots of oxygen-rich blood going to muscle fibers, it helps with osmosis, getting stiffness out of muscles by returning some of the water that's built up within each cell back into [the] bloodstream. Most people neglect this. A lot of coaches don't consider a hard interval set to be complete until their athletes have completed a recovery run within 12 hours of the workout. If you did the hard workout in the morning, do the recovery run in the afternoon. If you did it in the evening, do the recovery run the next morning.

Elite runner Nate Jenkins discovered for himself the benefit of active recovery. When he was running 100 miles per week in single sessions, he was able to build his volume all the way to 160 miles per week by adding a second run to his days. This second session was much slower than his typical 6- or 7-minute-per-mile training pace, usually constituting an additional 8 miles, but at an 8- or 9-minute-per-mile pace. "Then," Jenkins reflects, "I got greedy and tried to run a little bit less mileage, but doing those second runs at the normal training pace. I got run down very quickly and went back to the 100-mile week, but I still wasn't feeling right. I added back the eight-mile shakeout runs."

Such active recovery works for Jenkins, who prefers some kind of movement over complete rest. "With time completely off, your neuro-muscular system goes too far into rest and gets stiff," he says, suggesting a yoga session, core work, or a swim as good choices to keep the body moving while not taxing it further. U.S. Olympian Shalane Flanagan agrees: "I do a lot of hydrotherapy in general. When I'm feeling flat, I get in the pool."

WHAT MODALITY TO USE

Ultrarunner Annette Bednosky echoes Flanagan's statement on the benefits of swimming: "I have just started swimming and find the stretching out from swimming and then sitting in a hot tub is an excellent part of training. I am an icky swimmer, yet you don't have to be good at it to gain some of the benefits."

Using a different sport for active recovery can introduce not only variety of intensity but variety of muscle recruitment to your training. It can also provide a mental break for the single-sport athlete. However, Magill, as a running coach, suggests running as active recovery:

It all depends on what a person's goals are. If you want to become a better runner, I never suggest cross-training. If your goal is to stay active and fit, cross-training is a good thing to do. If you run a hard workout and do an easy bike ride for recovery, you're recruiting different muscle fibers.

Of course there's overlap, but you can't train to be a better runner by riding a bike. Exercise is cell-specific. You're training a different range of muscle fibers and separating the workload among different muscle fibers.

If you are a balanced runner capable of handling high mileage, running might make a fine active recovery workout for you—and running easy will contribute to your efficiency and positive adaptation to running's stresses. But if you have a history of injury or burnout, substituting a different modality for your active recovery session might work better. In each modality, the workout should be kept to 40 minutes or less; otherwise, it becomes an endurance workout rather than active recovery. Here are some options.

Swimming can be relaxing, especially once you have solid technique, and it works the body in a different relationship to gravity. The pressure of the water supports your muscles and facilitates recovery by helping remove edema, and the workout is, of course, nonimpact and engages your entire body—upper body, core, and lower body. If you want extra rest for your legs, you can swim with a pull buoy, which holds your legs up as you use your arms and core to swim. If you are a single-sport swimmer, include short, drill-based recovery workouts in your week.

Cycling is another nonimpact sport. Riding outdoors offers not only some active recovery time but also some sightseeing, either on the road or on a bike path or trail. (Mountain biking, however, may be too demanding to qualify as active recovery.) Riding indoors allows you to control the intensity completely. An easy ride on the bike trainer gives you time to catch a television show or movie and take a mental break, and it keeps you near your family, making it a good option for busy parents. Beware a group indoor cycling class, where you might be sucked into putting out an effort that's too hard to count as recovery. Cyclists should include one or more very easy recovery rides during the course of the week.

The elliptical trainer can be a good active recovery choice for runners because it mimics the running stride without the impact. (Multisport athletes will do better with an easy swim or bike ride, which gives them the active recovery workout while staying within their primary modalities.) You can also involve your upper body on the elliptical.

Like the elliptical trainer, easy running on a soft surface such as a cinder trail reduces the impact of running while going through the same range of motion. So does running in water, which can be done in shallow water or in deep water while wearing a flotation belt. It might look silly, but it's a fine workout. Another possibility is to run on an Alter-G treadmill, which reduces the runner's body weight by up to 80 percent. With the reduced body weight, athletes can expend much less energy—and receive much less impact—than on a regular treadmill or over-the-ground run.

Don't have access to a $75,000 Alter-G? Walking makes a fine recovery workout, and it can give you some quality time with a loved one—or your dog.

Whatever modality you choose, including easy efforts between your harder workouts will help both physiologically and psychologically. Your body will recover faster when you don't add heavy stress but, instead, move just enough to stimulate extra blood flow. And your mind will recover as well, by getting a break from the intensity of your moderate and harder workouts and, if you choose alternative sports for easy workouts, by getting a break from the routine of your usual activity.

QUICK TIPS

- Active recovery includes both a proper cooldown and stand-alone sessions of 20 to 40 minutes.
- The intensity of active recovery sessions should be very light—just enough to break a sweat.
- Including very easy days lessens the monotony of training and allows you to eke out more high-end efforts during your hard workouts.

7

Stress Reduction

Time: little	
Cost: low	
Accessibility: good	
Confidence: high	
Contraindications: none	

When you're wound tightly, for whatever reason, you don't get the downtime you need to bring your body into balance. Add this to the fatigue you're already carrying as a result of your training and it's a recipe for disaster. Have you ever noticed how poorly timed illness can be when you are building toward a big race? Have you become accident prone close to a major event? We often think of this as bad luck, but it can also be our bodies telling us—subtly or not—that we need a rest.

During my training for Ironman Coeur d'Alene 2009, I cut back on my writing and editing commitments so I could call training my work. Still, the work of training can be pretty intense, and I carried a heavy load of fatigue that manifested in a mental fog that thickened every time I approached a grocery store. I was unable to think beyond pizza.

My family ate a lot of pizza. One spring evening, I felt rested enough to make guacamole—a welcome break from pizza—and wound up in the emergency room after badly botching an avocado pit–removal trick using a butcher's knife. (The admitting nurse kindly suggested pit removal using a spoon next time.) The result was a row of stitches on my hand that kept me out of the water for a little more than a week. Two days after the cut, I made it through a century ride with my hand still in the hospital splint (an unforeseen benefit of aerobars). And the next weekend, stitches out prematurely, I raced a half-Iron-distance triathlon. Obviously, this was the peak of my training, and the various stressors in my life had conspired to make me clumsy.

The next year, training for the same race and on the same weekend, my yoga student Susan fell while climbing into her bathtub to soak her aching feet. A row of stitches patched up her eyebrow, which had made hard contact with the faucet head on her way down. Again, it was not coincidence; it was the workload catching up with her, and a little bad luck.

Removing life stress for even a few days can have a big effect on your performance. Elite runner Nate Jenkins tells the story of a running partner with a full plate who carried a lot of stress. This runner was expecting a child and buying a house while working full time and running 120 miles a week, "but not running that well," Jenkins says. "We went to Ireland for two races in four days. The first race, he was far and away the last [of the team]. We spent the next three days touring Ireland, eating, drinking, partying, not sleeping—burning the candle at both ends. In the second race, he was the first of us across the line by a good little bit. As poor preparation as that was for a race, that was easier than what he was doing at home!"

Finding ways to cope with both physical and psychological stress can help you integrate the work of training better, keeping you safer, more balanced, and more pleasant to be around. In this chapter, we'll take a big-picture view of stress.

PHYSICAL AND PSYCHOLOGICAL STRESS

Hans Selye, whose work marks the start of modern thinking on stress, subdivided stressors into eustress, or positive stress, and distress, or negative stress, as we saw in chapter 1. Physically, you need positive stress to create adaptations; psychologically, you need the challenge of positive stress to perform at your best. (Think of writing a term paper under deadline, delivering a speech, or running a race with big stakes.) When you can no longer adapt to and recover from the stress, however, it has become negative stress, which takes a toll on the body. Ultimately, your body can't distinguish between physical stress and mental stress, and it all becomes processed in the same way, with elevated cortisol and adrenaline levels; increased heart rate, blood pressure, and muscle tension; and a host of problems from stomach upset to headaches to trouble sleeping.

As athletes, we're familiar with physical stress, and we even actively seek it. This book aims to help you balance the physical stress you apply with careful attention to rest and recovery. But we must account for stressors from areas outside the physical since they will have a direct effect on your recovery.

Not all stress is bad. Sport psychologist Jack Raglin says, "A lot of people consider the stress of competition can be a source of stress that puts athletes over the edge. Our research contradicts that. Contrary to traditional beliefs, 30 to 45 percent of athletes require high levels of anxiety to perform best. Relaxation exercises for them can be counterproductive." An exception here is dwelling on the race and feeling signs of physical stress far from the race itself. However, in the few days leading up to the event, some anxiety is to be expected, and it can even help sharpen you for performance.

BE AWARE OF THE SOURCES OF YOUR STRESS

Psychological stress can come from your sport or from other areas of your life. We're used to the psychological stress before a race and the stress that accompanies workouts: the apprehension and fear of pain, the care that must be taken to be sure enough time is allotted for the workout and that equipment is lined up, the stress of working to achieve certain benchmarks in the workout, and the stress of missing them. But we sometimes fail to see how all our stressors—many of which come from far beyond the training hours—have a direct effect on our recovery and therefore on our training. And since the COVID-19 pandemic, with its shift to work-from-home setups and political discord, the amount of general stress has increased in addition to personal stressors. One 2012 study showed that life stress negatively impacted people's ability to recover from resistance training.[1]

All the various stressors in your life have a cumulative effect that you must keep in mind as you plan your training and recovery. When you have a big deadline at work, the extra stress will affect your training both directly and indirectly. In a direct manner, it may mean you have less mental energy for workouts or that you throw yourself into your intervals as a source of stress relief. Indirectly, you may be getting less sleep or spending more hours at your desk, which may bring with it tightness in your hip flexors, chest, shoulders, and neck, all of which can change your form in workouts. The stress of a move carries with it not only the emotional components but also the very real physical stress of packing, lifting heavy objects, climbing stairs repeatedly, bending over boxes to unpack, and the sundry other tasks that accompany the move. Pay attention to these conglomerate stressors and to how you respond to them.

A greater sense of awareness of your response will yield interesting insights into your behavior patterns, many of which will affect your recovery. When you are feeling anxious about something that appears to be out of your control, you may tend to control things you feel like you can control. For many athletes, that means training *more*. Say you couldn't make your target pace in a workout. This can create anxiety about your state of fitness, something you think you can control by repeating the workout the next day. Not so! Often, exactly what you need in such a situation is less work and more recovery.

FIND A BALANCE

Look for a balance between your commitments to your training, home life, and work life. There will be cycles and seasons in which one is more important than the others. The winter holidays are a time when your family may demand your focus. Depending on your job, there will be cyclical duties at work—the end of a fiscal year or college semester, the deadline for a major project. And your sport training probably falls into a season or two, with competitions grouped around a specific point on the calendar.

Mapping out these obligations can be very helpful as you work toward balance and stress reduction. Give this map the same care you would give your own annual training plan. Is there a period in the year when you'll be packing a child for a move to college? Note that. Is there a time when your partner has a particularly stressful work season? Note that. Travel both for work and for family should go on your list, too. Depending on how sophisticated you'd like to get, this map can be done with colored pens and paper, or it can be a spreadsheet or go right into a calendar application. How you do it isn't important. What matters is that you look at the big picture.

Sport psychologist Kate Hays had a patient who made just such a chart, creating a retrospective graph mapping the stressors in his work life versus his race times. He could then see, Hays says, "a direct connection between the high points of the stressful work season and poor times." Based on what he saw, he shifted his focus from triathlon to duathlon, quit his job, and took another job that didn't have such cyclically busy times.

While your own reaction might not be as drastic as changing sports and quitting your job, you will probably see some steps you can take to bring things more into balance. Coach Gordo Byrn advises, "If someone needs to crank their training stress up, the work stress needs to go down, and the family needs to buy in. Otherwise, there's disharmony in the athlete's life. You won't be able to recover when you're not meeting your obligations to your work and family."

Depending on the details of your home life, you might also need to schedule a period where you have greatly reduced stress. If you find time with your family relaxing, fantastic; if family time has its own stressors, be aware of that. The goal is not simply to replace stress from one area with stress from another. It is to give your system a chance to cycle between stress and rest, between work and recovery. Just as you get weekends off from work, you should get some time off from coping with stress—be it from training, your career, or your relationships.

MANAGING STRESS

Say No

Once you have a big-picture view of the stress in your life, you can work to find ways to reduce it. The number-one tool is learning the magic word: "No." So many of us are overcommitted, juggling dozens of obligations across the course of any given day. It can be incredibly tough to say no to an invitation to serve on a committee at work, to volunteer at your children's school, or to join a group for a ride. But often that is just what is needed so that you can best manage your other obligations without draining yourself completely.

I don't mean that you should say no to everything; in fact, that might encourage you to focus too obsessively on your training. Instead, prioritize. Choose only the most important commitments or those that give you the most joy or best use your talents and experience. When you are overcommitted, you're diluting the service you can offer others, because you are not fully present when you are not rested enough to focus on the task at hand or you are already thinking through what's next.

Make Space

Athletes are often busy people who perform at high levels in everything they do. It's crucial both for your recovery and for your overall well-being—as well as for your job performance—that you have plenty of space in your schedule for downtime and play. Matt Driller, PhD, is an associate professor in sport and exercise science at La Trobe University in Melbourne, and a senior recovery adviser at the Australian Institute of Sport, where he works across both Olympic and Paralympic sports. He says, "Most athletes I have worked with are incredibly busy people, so they often neglect to schedule time to just relax in their programs. I think the overall load (outside their training) can be ignored by most athletes and coaches. Spending time on their feet and rushing between commitments and appointments can take its toll on their overall recovery status."

Where can you make space in your schedule to do something that isn't directly related to your performance at work or in your sport? What other things do you enjoy that get you off your feet while putting you in nature, away from screens, and with people you love? Better yet, can you make space for unstructured time, free of goals? These downtime activities will directly contribute to your recovery, as well as making you a happier person who's more fun to be around.

Goal Check

In addition to having time for relaxing unconnected to your goals, having clear goals for your sport and your life is crucial. The construction of a good annual training plan starts with a goal-setting session. When you find yourself feeling stressed, return to those goals you have set. Ideally, you have goals that are reasonable, reachable, and quantifiable—that is, they follow the SMART acronym: specific, measurable, attainable, realistic, and time dependent. You probably also have goals for work and relationships, whether or not you have put them into words. Perhaps you are aiming for a promotion or to reach a sales figure. Perhaps you want to start your own company. Maybe you want to get married or have a child or send your child to college out of state. Each of these goals carries with it stress. Some of the stress is useful; much of it is not. When anxiety and a sense of being overwhelmed creep in, stop and reconsider your goals. Are your commitments in the service of your goals? If not, how can you change things? Sometimes doing this prompts you to revise your goal, which is good—the goal should not be set in stone.

When you are very clear on your goals, every decision is easier to make. You'll simply ask yourself this question: Does this choice align with my goals, or not? When you find it tough to make up your mind, revisit your goals; they may need some revision.

Think Ahead

As you realign your goals and prioritize what needs your attention, you might see things that you can do easily now to make things smoother down the road. For example, Jeff Brown, psychologist for the Boston Marathon (which runs the third week in April each year), suggests that runners get their taxes done early so that they can focus on relaxing before the trip to Boston. He sees timing as critical, especially when athletes travel for a peak event. "You don't want to get married two weeks after the marathon, or have some other major project," he says. "Those stressors may have an impact on performance, especially when juggling travel plans. Some athletes I've worked with simply overload themselves with travel, their marathon performance, sightseeing, and managing home from a distance. Focusing on the priority of the trip is key." Overextending yourself will interfere with your recovery at best and can lead to illness at worst.

Categorize

Before major races, I have my athletes fill out a detailed race plan. It helps them think ahead to manage their equipment, nutrition, and pacing. It also gives them a chance to state their race goals—a conservative goal, a stated goal, a radical goal, and a supersecret pie-in-the-sky goal. Defining these categories gives my athletes a chance to reflect on their training and their abilities under a range of race-day circumstances.

At the end of the race plan, I ask the athletes to make a list of their fears, worries, and concerns about the race. They then label these as either "in my control" or "out of my control" and write out a plan for how to cope should any of these fears come to pass. I've seen everything from sharks to flat tires to blisters to bad attitudes show up as fears, and I know from my athletes' feedback that simply naming these fears and creating a plan to deal with adverse conditions builds confidence and reduces stress.

Such listing isn't confined to a race plan. You can do the same thing for your life in general. Articulate what your fears are—writing them down is especially useful, as things often seem vastly less scary, even silly, when written down on paper—and categorize each as "in my control" or "out of my control." Construct a plan for dealing with the things that scare you, should they ever come to pass. You'll find this task helps you feel that you can handle almost everything that comes your way. Ultimately, one thing is always in your control, no matter how dire the situation: your attitude.

Process

Sport psychologist Danielle Adams Norenberg, head of performance psychology at the English Institute of Sport, suggests athletes take time for processing, both after the peak event of the season and throughout the training cycle. After a race performance, she suggests you make room to "be in the present moment in life—not necessarily anything to do with sport; ride the waves of emotions that inevitably come; and reconnect with friends, family, and perhaps nature, as well—which helps with being in the present moment." This is good advice not only for the postseason but also for in season. By planning an opportunity to decompress, Norenberg explains, you're creating space to "make sense of the emotions that came up in preparation and during [the event], to acknowledge, and to accept." Once you're familiar with this processing, she told me, you'll be able to weave it throughout the training cycle, so you have space for self-awareness in rest weeks, after big workouts, and ultimately every day (figure 7.1).

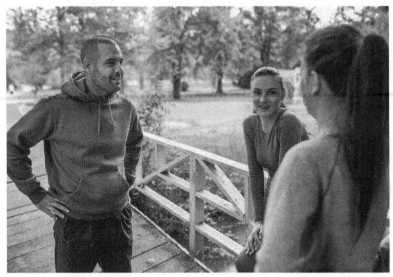

FIGURE 7.1
Talking through your experience with your peers and teammates is an important part of processing. *Getty Images/BjelicaS*

Relax

The restorative yoga poses and the meditation and breath-awareness exercises outlined in chapters 16 and 17 of this book will help you relax and recover from training stress. Beyond that, they will give you tools for coping when stress meets you in real life, whether it's the stress of a traffic jam, a major meeting, an argument with a loved one, or a race that's tough. In each of these situations, return to deep, full breaths, and relax everywhere you can, growing as efficient as possible by using energy only where it's needed. That might mean relaxing your jaw in traffic, your hands in the meeting, your shoulders in the argument, and all of the above in your race.

Get Help

A session or series of sessions with a counselor can teach you skills for managing stress and can go a long way toward helping you put your goals in perspective. A sports psychologist can help you with this, and, frankly, visiting a sports psychologist may be easier to wrap your brain around than visiting a general clinician. The rise of telehealth options means that you might be able to find a specialist in your unique area of competition, or who has life experiences similar to yours.

Depending on your needs, your sports psychologist can teach you mental skills for competition and for life in general. Psychotherapist Marv Zauderer says, "When I work with athletes on goal setting, I'm not just working on goals for things you want to achieve in your sport. Goals can help you put sport in the right place in your life." Doing so creates a healthy balance among training, work, and relationships.

QUICK TIPS

- Take a look at the big picture of your year, marking stressful times during your training, work, and family life.
- Manage your stressors by learning to say no to projects that spread you too thin.
- Have a clear sense of your goals and come back to them often.

8

Sleep

> **Time:** little to moderate
>
> **Cost:** free
>
> **Accessibility:** high
>
> **Confidence:** high
>
> **Contraindications:** none

One of my coaching clients, Tara, has a strict rule on sleep. If she doesn't get six hours of sleep in the night, she won't run the next day, reasoning that running tired does more harm than good. This is a fantastic policy to implement because, the truth is, many of us try to get by on far too little sleep. As physical therapist Brian Beatty says, "Most people's recovery plan is five hours of sleep and a lot of coffee." But as coach Matt Dixon points out: "Sleep is your number one, completely legal, and completely free performance enhancer for sport and for life."

Your sleep affects not just your recovery but also your ability to perform to your potential in workouts. When you don't get adequate sleep, your motor response is dulled, which can compromise your form or ingrain inefficient neuromuscular patterns—bad habits. Research at

Stanford University shows that athletes who get plenty of sleep demonstrate improved ability at sprinting, faster reaction times, and improved moods.[1] Anecdotal evidence bears this out. Retired elite runner Tera Moody, who has a history of insomnia, finds that sleep is crucial to her recovery. "When I get nine hours of sleep, I feel like Superwoman and my workouts are amazing," she says. "If I'm not sleeping well, I have to take extra recovery days between workouts and everything feels a lot harder."

There are further implications for athletes of the importance of sleep: Karine Spiegel and colleagues have shown that even a week of curtailed sleep causes adverse effects on glucose uptake and cortisol levels (engaging the sympathetic nervous system).[2] If your glucose uptake is inhibited, you are less able to refuel before, during, and after your workouts. While research into the precise effect of sleep on athletic recovery continues, there is agreement among athletes, coaches, and physiologists that sleep matters. You'll need to pay attention to your own sleep habits to determine what is the optimal amount for you.

Because disturbed sleep can be a strong indicator of overtraining, it's critical to keep an eye on your sleep habits. It might mean tracking the number of hours you sleep as well as the quality of your sleep, and you might also note how alert you feel during the day. If you see a deterioration, set aside time to repay your sleep debt, dropping a workout or two if necessary so you can sleep in.

WHAT HAPPENS DURING SLEEP

As you sleep, you progress through four stages: three non–rapid eye movement (NREM) stages, and one rapid eye movement stage (REM sleep). Stage NREM1, light sleep, involves a relaxation of your muscles and slowing eye movements—it's the period in which you drift into and out of sleep. In stage NREM2, your eyes stop moving, and your brain waves slow. Stage NREM3 includes the very slow brain waves called delta waves; you are in deep sleep. Your endocrine system releases hormones, including growth hormone, which are critical to your adaptation to training. REM is the fourth stage, often coming 70 to 90

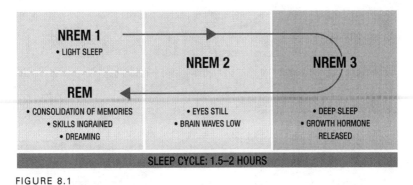

FIGURE 8.1
Stages of sleep
Note: The figure shows one complete sleep cycle. The cycle continues through the night.

minutes into the cycle. During this period, you consolidate memories and ingrain skills, which is obviously important for your athletic performance. A full cycle takes an hour and a half to two hours and then repeats NREM2, NREM3, and REM sleep (figure 8.1). As the night wears on, the amount of REM sleep increases, and the time spent in stage NREM3 decreases. We need adequate amounts of all types of sleep to function well and to recover fully.

HOW MUCH SLEEP TO GET

In an ideal world, you'd fall asleep about 20 minutes after climbing into bed. Nodding off quicker can be a sign of sleep debt. Then, ideally, you'd sleep until you were done sleeping, which we sometimes call being "slept out." For many people, this will be slightly more than eight hours per night, enough to let you wake up without needing an alarm. If you do not get enough sleep each night, you'll accrue "sleep debt," for which your body will eventually demand repayment. Plentiful sleep should be a key feature of your recovery plan.

In times of heavy training, be sure to block off extra time for sleep as part of your stress-management plan, in which you balance your obligations to work, family, and training. When training is heavy, ideally your workload will be lighter, and your family will understand your need for more sleep. One conventional rule of thumb, especially useful for runners, will help you get a sense of what works: If you are running 60 miles a week, you should aim to get an extra 60 minutes of sleep each day. Expressed in time units, if you're training 10 hours a week, an extra hour of sleep daily should improve your recovery. Likewise, if you're training 15 hours a week, an hour and a half is in order; a load of 20 hours a week would suggest you get two hours beyond the standard eight. While increasing sleep this much may not be realistic, it does encourage you to value sleep.

NAPPING

My former coach, Joan Nesbit Mabe, ran the 10,000 meters at the 1996 Olympics. She has long had a daily napping ritual, which she thinks made a big difference in her ability to recover and to fit 12 workouts into the week during her days as an elite runner. "That's twelve work days with only seven nights to sleep," she says. "I used napping to collapse twelve days into seven, kind of like the tesseract in *A Wrinkle in Time*. Every workout was preceded by sleep, be it a full night's sleep or an afternoon power nap. I never saw sleeping as lazy, but smart—and sort of sneaky, because I found a way to speed recovery without using performance-enhancing drugs."

A 2022 meta-analysis of sleep studies on napping shows that a nap of 30–60 minutes improved performance, both cognitive and physical, and reduced the perception of fatigue.[3] Athletes performed best when they waited more than an hour after the nap to train.

Depending on the amount of time you have—and whether you are carrying any sleep debt—the length of your nap may vary. A short nap—say, 20 minutes—will give you a period of NREM2 sleep, while a longer nap of an hour and a half or more can take you through the REM cycle. There is a period between the shorter and longer nap, somewhere around 45 minutes of sleep, in which you can find yourself waking groggier than you were when you started, so plan ahead when you lie down. If you can get into the habit of napping, you'll learn what the best parameters are for you. Notice also when your body feels ready to nap. Depending on your own circadian rhythm, you might find early or mid-afternoon the best time for a rest. Don't let your nap grow so long that you can't drift off easily at bedtime.

HOW TRAVEL AFFECTS SLEEP

Travel affects sleep habits, especially if you move across time zones. The change in environment alone can keep you awake or disturb your sleep, and that's compounded when your internal clock doesn't mesh with the time at your destination. Do what you can to create a restful environment for sleep (as outlined later in the chapter), and be sure you head into any travel, especially travel for a race, as well rested as possible.

Moving across time zones, figure that you'll need a day per time zone to adapt. If you're traveling from the East Coast to the West Coast of the United States for a race, or from the West Coast to Hawaii, arriving three days early would be a good plan. Westward travel is easier because you won't have to wake up any earlier than usual. Traveling east, conversely, is harder on the body, as you'll need to wake up earlier than you're used to. Opening the blinds and getting sunlight will help you adapt by resetting your internal clock (figure 8.2).

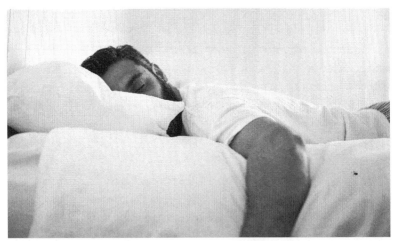

FIGURE 8.2
Sleep is one of your most powerful tools for recovery. *Getty Images/laflor*

SLEEP TRACKERS

The rise of wearable technology means that athletes have a range of tools available to help them measure sleep. But you should consider three things before putting too much stock in your technology to track your sleep.

First, simply tracking sleep—or having the tools to do it—doesn't mean you'll sleep better. In fact, it might mean you'll sleep worse, if you start to obsess over the numbers, a condition called orthosomnia. Worrying about not sleeping is a surefire way not to sleep! As sleep specialist Dr. Matt Driller, who has done extensive research on sleep and athletic recovery,[4] told me, "Sleep monitors are just a tool." He says athletes expecting the simple presence of a tracker to improve sleep "is like buying a bathroom scale and expecting to lose weight. They only work if they inform changes to behavior."

Second, your tracker may not be measuring correctly. Depending on a range of factors, including your skin tone, whether you share your bed, how frequently your tracker retrieves data, and which data it measures, it may credit you for sleep when you were lying in bed reading—or lying in bed unmoving, but wide awake. In experimenting with an Oura ring for sleep tracking, I quickly realized that if I donned the ring when I got into bed to read—a period that, depending on how exciting the book is and how sleepy I am, might last from 10 minutes to an hour—my data would look like I had trouble falling asleep. Now I put the ring on at lights out, which means that my "latency"—the amount of time it takes for me to fall asleep once the tracker recognizes I am lying down—is skewed in the other direction, sometimes as little as 3 minutes.

Third, your own perception of how well you slept will affect your performance and behavior regardless of how much you *actually* slept. Multiple studies have shown that placebo sleep—that is, being told that they slept more or better than they did—led participants to perform better on tests.[5] And telling people they slept worse than they did had the opposite effect.[6] With that much wiggle room, be sure to take the data from your tracker with a grain of salt.

ALCOHOL AND YOUR SLEEP

If you start using a sleep tracker and you sometimes consume alcohol, you will very quickly see in your data the correlation between having a few drinks and the quality of your sleep. Alcohol, especially when consumed close to bedtime and/or with a later dinner, will show up in your sleep data. It delays the lowering of your resting heart rate and adversely affects the quality of your sleep. Coach Matt Dixon explains this is one of the major arguments for tracking your data. "It's been really useful—for myself, included," he told me. "I really like beer and I'm English, and I don't want to give it up. I don't want to become evangelical, but I've shifted to nonalcoholic beer during the week. Luckily enough, there's loads of really good nonalcoholic beers. I just realized [from sleep tracking] that's going to have a major impact on my performance."

SETTING UP BETTER SLEEP

Keeping a routine will help you regulate your sleep better. Aim to get to bed at the same time every night and to wake up around the same time every morning. This holds true on weekends, as well. Your bedroom should be quiet, cool, and dark and used not as a den for reading and watching television but as a sanctuary for sleep.

What you do in the few hours before sleep affects your ability to unwind and to stay asleep. If you have a late-day workout, don't let it creep too close to bedtime so that you aren't still jacked up when it's time to lie down. Avoid caffeine after lunchtime; its effects can linger for hours. And even though drinking alcohol might help you feel relaxed or drowsy, it will likely interfere with the quality of your sleep and isn't a great strategy for getting quality rest.

A relaxing unwinding ritual can help prepare you for bed. Take the half hour before you get in bed to enjoy a cup of herbal tea (chamomile is a traditional choice, considered soporific), soak in a warm bath (perhaps with Epsom salts; see chapter 12), do a few restorative yoga poses (see chapter 16), or focus on your breathing and meditate (chapter 17). Exactly what you do is less important than the ceremony of doing it. In time, you'll associate this ritual with bedtime, and it will cue you to fall asleep.

Whether or not you notice that light affects your sleep, using a sleep mask has been shown to help with performance and alertness the next day.[7] The right mask will also send a signal to your body that it's time for sleep. Unsolicited endorsement: I've experimented with dozens of mask options and have found the Manta sleep mask far and away the best. It has repositionable memory-foam "doughnuts" that circle your eyes to block out all light without crushing your eyelashes.

If you have trouble sleeping and are considering using sleep aids—even melatonin, sold as a dietary supplement—talk to your health care provider and, if you have one, your coach. You'll want to check that any substance you're considering taking is both safe for you and not a banned substance on the World Anti-Doping Agency's (WADA) list. Your coach should hear about your sleeping problems, too, because they may be a sign that you are carrying too heavy a training load. Tweaking your training plan can help you balance work and rest.

Reducing life stress will also help you sleep. See chapter 7 for more on stress reduction.

QUICK TIPS

- Getting enough sleep is crucial to athletic performance.
- Sleep until you wake up satisfied, without an alarm—this might mean nine hours or even more per night.
- Naps supplement your nighttime sleep and help reduce your sleep debt.
- An evening ritual can help you settle down for sleep.

9

Nutrition and Hydration

Time: little to moderate

Cost: low to moderate

Accessibility: good

Confidence: high

Contraindications: food allergies may limit your choices

After my first marathon, I couldn't eat normally. The nausea that was my constant companion stayed with me a full two days, forcing me to cancel my post-race dinner reservations and making what would have been an indulgent room service meal completely unpalatable. An hour after finishing my first Ironman, however, I was happily eating and sipping champagne. The difference? I'd figured out fueling *during* the race, to the benefit of my post-race recovery. As you may know well from personal experience, the right nutrition can make or break your race. The longer the event, the more crucial it is to figure out how to eat during the race. But that's only part of the puzzle. You also need to learn the best ways to fuel your recovery so that you are ready for the next training session.

Proper recovery nutrition happens not simply in the immediate postworkout period, but all the time. We hear a lot about the "glycogen synthesis window," or the recovery window, which is open widest in the first two hours after exercise, and a good recovery nutrition plan will certainly address that time. But nutrition for recovery extends far beyond this window; it happens all day, day in and day out.

DAILY EATING

Your best approach to recovery nutrition is, quite simply, to eat well all the time. A healthy diet, states Michael Pollan in his now-famous manifesto from *In Defense of Food*, is composed of "food. Not too much. Mostly plants."[1] A wide variety of brightly colored foods, mostly vegetables and fruits and, whenever possible, organic and locally sourced, will provide you with most of what you need. Prepackaged and processed foods—the bars, gels, and powdered drinks that line the shelves of any athlete's pantry—have their place, but it is a limited place and pertains to the time immediately preceding, during, and sometimes after exercise. Even then, real food is often the better option, depending on the individual's constitution and the intensity and duration of exercise. For specific guidelines on how to fuel during and refuel after exercise, consult the International Society of Sports Nutrition guidelines on nutrient timing, which address a range of scenarios.[2]

Performance nutrition coach Scott Tindal, cofounder of Fuelin, explains of nutrition: "It's not sexy. There are some sexy elements about it, but the reality is eating five to seven servings of fruit and vegetables daily combined with good quality dietary proteins—lean proteins—and keeping your fats to sources that are predominantly monounsaturated fats, in the form of sources like olive oils, almonds, avocados, and omega-3s through food and supplementation (when required): that's what will make the real difference. It is all about making sure that the fuel you are providing your body with is commensurate to your activity levels and desired purpose." Your daily diet should include a good balance of macronutrients (carbohydrates, protein, and fats). The precise proportion of each that works best depends on your constitution, sport, and activity level and must be determined individually. Consult with a registered dietician specializing in sports nutrition if you need advice. This is one of the best uses of your recovery budget! While we often get into a habit of eating the same thing day in and day out, and while it can be easy to have a weekly schedule (Wednesday night is pizza night), variety ensures we get the most from our food. In chapter 4, we saw the strain of a monotonous training load; don't get so mired in habit that you have a monotonous diet.

Not only should you eat a variety of foods, but you should eat them in sufficient amounts to ensure you have energy for your training, your recovery, and your daily life. Remember, RED-S, relative energy deficiency in sport, can affect athletes of any gender and level of experience. Happily, paying attention to your recovery will help you tune in to whether you are providing your system enough energy to cover all your commitments.

Eating a well-rounded, natural diet will provide your body with the elements it needs to recover: carbohydrates to supply and replenish energy in the form of glycogen, protein to deliver amino acids to rebuild muscle fiber, and fats to insulate the body and to carry vitamins to the cells. Fall short on any of these and you'll be shortchanging your recovery (figure 9.1).

THE RECOVERY SNACK OR MEAL

The importance of the recovery snack—food eaten shortly after a workout, and outside of regular meal times—depends on the context of your training. If you've finished a moderate-intensity run and won't do another moderate or hard workout for two days, you'll probably get the nutrients you need for recovery from your regular meals, which is why I call it a "snack or meal." If, however, you've finished a three-hour ride in the morning and have an evening run planned, the recovery snack and its timing become much more important—but they may actually be lunch, not a "snack" per se. Likewise, if you've finished your peak event for the season and are heading into a transition period with no

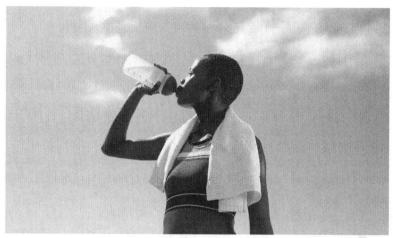

FIGURE 9.1
Aim to take in approximately 150 percent of your fluid losses. *Getty Images/
jacoblund*

organized training, a recovery snack is not critical. But if you've finished
a long run and have depleted your glycogen stores, you need to pay attention to getting a recovery snack quickly, even outside of regular meal
times, so that you can restock for the next week of training.

Recovery Nutrition Starts Early

Your recovery nutrition actually begins *before* your workout. You'll
need to check that you are entering the workout with a full tank, so to
speak. While you may not have full glycogen stores, you'll want to have
enough energy to complete the workout: Ideally, you'll approach the
workout with a plan that trains your body to use the energy sources
you'll need in your race—fat for endurance workouts, glycogen for
higher-intensity efforts. Starting your workout with a deficit will interfere with your recovery.

Likewise, take in fluid and carbohydrates if your workout is a long
one. Doing so will ensure that you don't create a massive deficit,
which will be harder to overcome and will interfere with your recovery. When you deplete your glycogen supply, you hit the dreaded

wall—a condition that can jettison your race. Beyond that, it may take a number of days to replenish your glycogen stores.

Timing of the Recovery Snack or Meal

The carbohydrates you consume in the first 30 minutes after exercise will lead to higher glycogen levels than if you wait for two hours after the workout to begin eating again.[3] For this reason, we often hear about a "glycogen window," in which we have to take in our recovery snack for maximum benefits. And while that's true, it's not as hard and fast as some would make it seem. The window doesn't slam shut at 30 minutes postexercise. You have two hours after your workout when you can take in that recovery snack. But you'll still be replenishing glycogen depleted during a morning workout when you eat your lunch, your afternoon snack, and your dinner. In fact, if you're more depleted, you'll still be replenishing your glycogen stores the next day. Don't get too hung up on the 30-minute rule, but do remember to pay attention to your recovery snack after longer or intense workouts when you need to recover quickly.

Composition of the Recovery Snack or Meal

Your recovery snack should be a mixture of fluids, sodium, carbohydrates, protein, and not too much fat. Fat can interfere with your body's ability to process the carbohydrates and protein in your recovery snack. Here's a look at the breakdown.

Fluids

The recovery snack or meal needs to include fluid to help offset the fluid lost during your workout. How will you know how much you've lost? By weighing yourself pre- and postworkout, ideally nude so that your wet clothing doesn't skew the postworkout measurement. You don't need to do this for every single workout, but an occasional weigh-in before and after your longer or harder workouts will show you how much water weight you're losing.

You'll need to replace most of each pound—or 16 ounces—of fluid you've lost. The American Dietetic Association (ADA) suggests you drink from 16 to 24 ounces for every pound of weight lost during the workout. Hitting the higher end of this range, 24 ounces per pound lost, accounts for losses through respiration, perspiration, and urination. Paying attention to fluids will help you rehydrate more quickly and set you up for your next training session. See the "Hydration" section later in the chapter.

Sodium

Even if you are a so-called salty sweater, the concentration of sodium in your blood actually increases during your workout, because you lose far more fluid than sodium as you sweat. But this loss of sodium needs to be offset by taking in sodium after your training session so you can restore your preworkout balance. It can come from a sports drink, but many sports drinks don't have enough sodium (see table 9.1). You can supplement by using table salt as part of your recovery snack or by taking salt tablets or electrolyte capsules. Sodium pulls glucose and water into your cells, so it's important that you get your sodium stores refilled.

Table 9.1.   Sodium in beverages (8 oz.)

BEVERAGE	SODIUM
Swanson vegetable broth	940 mg
Swanson chicken broth	860 mg
V-8 juice	675 mg
Tomato juice	650 mg
Gatorade Endurance	200 mg
Power Bar Endurance	190 mg
Starbucks Dark Chocolate Mocha Frappuccino	160 mg
Chocolate milk	150 mg
Milk	125 mg
Club soda	75 mg
Coca-Cola	30 mg
Diet Coke	26 mg
Hammer HEED	20 mg

Carbohydrates

Your recovery snack or meal should contain somewhere between 1.0 and 1.5 grams of carbohydrates per kilogram of your body weight, with 1.2 grams per kilogram of body weight a common target. (To figure your weight in kilos, divide your weight in pounds by 2.2.) That's roughly the equivalent of 0.5 grams of carbohydrates per pound of body weight. Each gram of carbohydrates contains 4 calories. To make things easy, see table 9.2 for your target range of carbohydrates to consume in the recovery snack.

Table 9.2.   Carbohydrates (CHO) for recovery snack

BODY WEIGHT IN KILOGRAMS	BODY WEIGHT IN POUNDS	1.0 G OF CHO PER KILO	1.2 G OF CHO PER KILO	1.5 G OF CHO PER KILO	1.0 G OF CHO PER KILO IN CALORIES	1.2 G OF CHO PER KILO IN CALORIES	1.5 G OF CHO PER KILO IN CALORIES
45.5	100	45.5	54.5	68.2	181.8	218.2	272.7
47.7	105	47.7	57.3	71.6	190.9	229.1	286.4
50.0	110	50.0	60.0	75.0	200.0	240.0	300.0
52.3	115	52.3	62.7	78.4	209.1	250.9	313.6
54.5	120	54.5	65.5	81.8	218.2	261.8	327.3
56.8	125	56.8	68.2	85.2	227.3	272.7	340.9
59.1	130	59.1	70.9	88.6	236.4	283.6	354.5
61.4	135	61.4	73.6	92.0	245.5	294.5	368.2
63.6	140	63.6	76.4	95.5	254.5	305.5	381.8
65.9	145	65.9	79.1	98.9	263.6	316.4	395.5
68.2	150	68.2	81.8	102.3	272.7	327.3	409.1
70.5	155	70.5	84.5	105.7	281.8	338.2	422.7
72.7	160	72.7	87.3	109.1	290.9	349.1	436.4
75.0	165	75.0	90.0	112.5	300.0	360.0	450.0
77.3	170	77.3	92.7	115.9	309.1	370.9	463.6
79.5	175	79.5	95.5	119.3	318.2	381.8	477.3
81.8	180	81.8	98.2	122.7	327.3	392.7	490.9
84.1	185	84.1	100.9	126.1	336.4	403.6	504.5
86.4	190	86.4	103.6	129.5	345.5	414.5	518.2
88.6	195	88.6	106.4	133.0	354.5	425.5	531.8
90.9	200	90.9	109.1	136.4	363.6	436.4	545.5
93.2	205	93.2	111.8	139.8	372.7	447.3	559.1
95.5	210	95.5	114.5	143.2	381.8	458.2	572.7
97.7	215	97.7	117.3	146.6	390.9	469.1	586.4
100.0	220	100.0	120.0	150.0	400.0	480.0	600.0
102.3	225	102.3	122.7	153.4	409.1	490.9	613.6
104.5	230	104.5	125.5	156.8	418.2	501.8	627.3
106.8	235	106.8	128.2	160.2	427.3	512.7	640.9
109.1	240	109.1	130.9	163.6	436.4	523.6	654.5
111.4	245	111.4	133.6	167.0	445.4	534.5	668.2
113.6	250	113.6	136.4	170.5	454.5	545.5	681.8

As you can see, that's a decent amount of calories. You'll be taking them in after a workout of 90 minutes or longer, though, and you must think of them as crucial to your recovery, because replenishing the glycogen stores you've just depleted is a prerequisite for your next workout to have any quality effect.

Protein

The traditional recommendation for protein in the recovery meal or snack has been 20 grams. It can come from soy; whey; pulses like beans, lentils, or peas; fish; or a lean meat source. Performance nutrition coach Scott Tindal explains that even more protein is required in this postworkout feed: 30 to 40 grams, aiming for a total of 1.6 to 2.5 grams of protein per kilogram of body weight daily. That range equates to 86 to 135 grams of protein daily for a 120-pound athlete, and 144 to 225 grams of protein daily for a 200-pound athlete. Tindal would recommend a minimum intake of 120 grams of protein for athletes who weigh 120 pounds (55 kilograms) or less.

Coach Matt Dixon concurs. He explains that most of the athletes he sees coming into endurance sports are undereating relative to their training demands. Rather than this being a question of body image, he says it's "people just not having the appreciation of the amount of calories required to facilitate consistent training demands and optimal recovery. The vast majority—90 percent of athletes—are underconsuming, particularly around protein." Remember: consulting with a sports nutritionist is one of the best uses of your recovery budget.

Recovery Snack Options

Chocolate milk has been promoted as an ideal recovery drink ever since a 2006 study (funded, in part, by the dairy industry) showed that it aided recovery as well as or better than the commercial products Gatorade and Endurox R-4.[4] It can be a very palatable choice, especially after a very long or intense workout because you might not have much of an appetite. This is when a liquid snack is most appealing.

For convenience, you might choose a preformulated recovery drink or recovery bar, and that's fine. When you can, however, aim to prepare your own recovery snack. It gives you a chance to control the ingredients, to include organic and locally sourced items whenever possible, and to customize the flavor and texture to please your palate.

Examples of a suitable recovery snack:

- Chocolate milk
- Chocolate soymilk
- Bagel with jam, cream cheese, peanut butter, or a slice of turkey
- Smoothie (fruit and/or vegetables blended with cow's milk; soy, almond, or rice milk; or yogurt)
- Fruit and yogurt
- Cereal with cow's milk or soy, almond, or rice milk
- Fresh juice and a handful of nuts

With any of these snacks, include water or sports drink to rehydrate you and consider adding salt or supplementing with electrolytes.

Beyond the Recovery Snack

Your recovery continues well beyond the recovery snack. You'll do well to take in another 1.0 to 1.2 grams of carbohydrates per kilogram of body weight about two hours after your recovery snack. This often comes at a regular mealtime—lunch after a morning workout, dinner after an afternoon or all-day session—so it can be composed of real, whole foods. Beyond that meal, pay attention to the amount of carbohydrates you're consuming for the rest of the day and be sure to take in protein and fat, as well.

Eating to Reduce Inflammation

While some inflammation is a normal product of training, carrying too much inflammation may aggravate overuse patterns, leading to injury, and may contribute not only to inflammatory diseases such as arthritis and lupus but also to heart disease, some cancers, and Alzheimer's. What you eat can affect your body's inflammatory response. Certain foods can help your body combat inflammation: berries, rich in phytochemicals and antioxidants; cold-water fish, such as salmon and mackerel, as well as walnuts and flaxseed, all of which are rich in omega-3 fatty acids; spices such as ginger and garlic; and coffee and tea. A healthy, Mediterranean-influenced diet high in vegetables, beans, fish, and olive oil works well.

Many books and websites offer details on an anti-inflammatory diet. It's worth looking into because such diets emphasize whole grains, beans, healthy fats, and plenty of produce, which is a great diet for athletes, regardless of its anti-inflammatory properties.

During periods of heavy training, take special care to avoid junk food and foods high in saturated fat and sugar. (Of course, this is a good policy year-round.) Our Western diets are generally too heavy in omega-6 fatty acids, which feed hormones that promote inflammation, and often too low in omega-3s, which do the opposite. Polyunsaturated vegetable oils, found in most processed foods, are a source of omega-6s. While we need both omega-3 and omega-6 fatty acids, we need them in the correct ratio—pretty much as low as we can get it toward 2 to 1, or even 1 to 1. For more on omega-3 fatty acids, see chapter 10, on supplements, but aim to get most of your nutritional needs from food instead of supplements.

HYDRATION

It's critical to your performance and your recovery to stay hydrated. Just as good nutrition throughout the day is key, your hydration for recovery starts even before your workout. That usually doesn't mean you need to prehydrate in huge amounts—especially as that fluid will often pass right through you, taking sodium with it. Instead, maintain a decent state of hydration throughout your day.

While dehydration is a natural effect that occurs during training and racing, if you get too deep into dehydration, your performance suffers—and worse, with it your judgment about the timing of your fluid intake. When you become dehydrated, your heart rate rises to pump the smaller volume of blood to your working muscles. Your effort feels harder. You can develop gastrointestinal problems. None of these symptoms aid peak performance! If you do more than one workout in a day, or if any of your workouts take place in the heat, you need to pay special attention to the amount of fluid you're consuming.

One way to be sure you're not jettisoning your ability to recover by underhydrating is to weigh yourself before and after a workout. Nude is best—take off your wet workout clothes, lest they inflate the number after your workout. Sports scientist Andy Blow, cofounder of Precision Hydration, explains that a loss of 1–3 percent of your body weight during the course of a workout is expected, and will probably be replaced as you simply drink to your thirst. But losing more than that is a sign that you may need to work on your hydration during the workout, so that you don't have a big deficit to overcome before your next training session.

To be sure you aren't hampering your recovery, aim to take in approximately 150 percent of your losses from during the workout, Blow suggests. The excess 50 percent beyond your losses covers the loss from breathing, sweating, and urinating. This rule of thumb should carry through most moderate workouts done in cold or cooler conditions. For workouts in hot or humid conditions—especially if you aren't acclimated to the temperature and humidity—or for multiple workouts done in a day, you'll need to pay more careful attention to your hydration for recovery, and include some sodium in or with fluids, as this is proven to increase the restoration of plasma.[5] Blow explains, "If you don't rehydrate quite proactively and aggressively after the first session, you might perform okay in the second session, but then you're almost certainly going to get up on the back foot the next day." This can lead to a negative trend.

Aside from noting weight deviations from your baseline, the easiest way to determine your state of hydration is by checking the color of your urine. It should be light colored or almost clear. Yellow or brown urine indicates dehydration. (Note that some vitamin supplements will give your urine a bright yellow hue.)

The best beverages to replace fluids lost in training and racing will include some sodium to encourage the body to retain these fluids for use in rehydration, as covered earlier. If you are drinking water, be sure to have some saltier food alongside it. Straight water is often passed through the body quickly and released as urine. And drinking too much plain water in order to stick to a predetermined schedule can lead to hyponatremia, an imbalance between sodium and fluid levels that can cause serious problems, even death. You might choose instead a sports drink with sodium, chicken or vegetable broth, tomato juice, or a home-made smoothie with some added salt. Some bodies don't need much sodium to replenish sweat losses; others need a lot. Exactly the right amount of sodium replenishment for your body depends on where you fall on the spectrum. If you find you're regularly losing a lot of weight in your longer or hotter workouts, you may want to have a sweat test and consult with an expert on a hydration plan to support your unique needs for training and recovering well. The information at the Precision Hydration website (precisionhydration.com) is one good place to start.

Paying close attention to your nutrition and hydration will ensure you're fueling your body with everything it needs to recover properly (figure 9.2).

Postworkout Timing

Here's a timeline for your postworkout nutrition after a long (more than 90 minutes) or very hard workout.

- Within about 30 minutes: Consume a recovery snack to give you the carbohydrates, protein, and sodium you need, according to the tables in this chapter; drink to your thirst.
- Within about two hours: Enjoy a balanced meal; drink to your thirst.
- For the rest of the day: Continue drinking to your thirst and eating a variety of healthy foods.

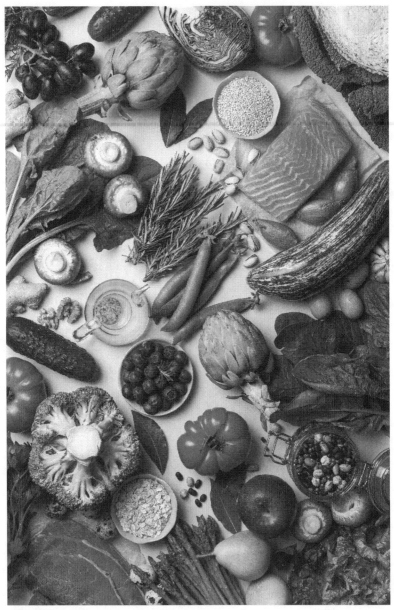

FIGURE 9.2
Your diet should include a rainbow's worth of colors. *Getty Images/Aamulya*

Protein and the Vegetarian

If you are a vegetarian or vegan eater, you'll need to pay extra attention to your protein intake. Plant proteins aren't digested in the same amount as animal proteins, so the American Dietetic Association suggests vegetarian athletes eat 10 percent more protein than those who eat meat. The rule of thumb is then 1.3 to 1.8 grams per kilogram of body weight per day.

Vegetarian athletes must also be careful to consume enough calcium, iron, zinc, riboflavin, and vitamins B-12 and D. If you follow a vegetarian or vegan diet and feel you're having trouble recovering between workouts, it's a good idea to ask a sports dietician to analyze your diet and help you get enough nutrients.

Alcohol

Consumed in moderation, alcohol can be a pleasurable part of your weekly diet. Beyond a drink or two, however, alcohol will quickly begin to interfere with your recovery, including the replenishment of your glycogen stores, so consider its place in your day-to-day routine. In addition, if you find yourself turning to alcohol for stress reduction, consider your priorities and goals. Are you making the healthiest choices? Do they support your big-picture goals? Just as spot-icing a certain body part or turning to supplements should send up a red flag, so should relying on alcohol as part of your daily diet.

QUICK TIPS

- Recovery nutrition is, quite simply, good nutrition all the time.
- Emphasize variety in your diet.
- A balanced diet can help combat systemic inflammation and lower your recovery times.
- Stay hydrated, during exercise and all day.

Supplements

Time: little

Cost: moderate

Accessibility: good

Confidence: depends on supplement

Contraindications: sensitivity to supplements; for athletes subject to drug testing, possible contamination

Supplements are designed to cover deficiencies in your diet. If you eat a varied, healthy diet rich in fruits, vegetables, whole grains, and lean protein, you should be setting yourself up for maximum recovery. (If you are unsure about whether you're eating right, have a sports nutritionist analyze your diet.) But beyond whole-foods nutrition, a few supplements may enhance your recovery. In this chapter, we'll look at the most beneficial supplements, as well as things you might be using now that aren't worth your time and money—or, in the case of nonsteroidal anti-inflammatory drugs (NSAIDs), can even compromise your health.

If you are accustomed to supplementing, it may have been a while since you gave thought to what you are taking and why. Because reducing stress and simplifying your life will help your recovery, spend a moment considering why you use each supplement in your arsenal, whether it's working for you, what its drawbacks might be (whether in pricing, maintenance, or system upset), and how it serves your athletic and personal goals. You might find a simpler regimen works just as well, or you might recommit to your current choices. Just be sure you are not using something from a bottle to counter the effects of too little sleep and too much stress.

Supplements are not subject to Food and Drug Administration (FDA) approval. Many have not undergone the rigorous clinical testing required for FDA-approved drugs, and producers are not required to substantiate their claims about their products' effectiveness. Supplement production is not regulated with federal oversight, so contamination is always possible. As a competitive athlete, you are ultimately responsible for what you ingest, and if you are subject to World Anti-Doping Agency (WADA) drug testing, you must be particularly rigorous and careful about what you allow to cross your lips (or your skin, if you use topical creams and balms). It's best to talk to your coach and your health care providers—including your sports nutritionist—before using any of the supplements described here.

TAKE A SKEPTIC'S APPROACH

Nick Tiller, PhD, outlines smart, research-informed ways to evaluate grand claims in his 2020 book *The Skeptic's Guide to Sports Science*.[1] He explains that it's tempting to believe in a simple solution to a complex problem—to spend a little money on a supplement, or a massage device—while ignoring the fundamentals that actually help your recovery and your whole system: sleep, solid nutrition, and stress management. Supplements in particular prey on this desire for a quick fix. He describes his process of evaluating claims:

> Okay, you're telling me that it works. You've got to convince me—and as a scientist and as a skeptic, I'm open-minded but quite difficult to convince.

As Carl Sagan's famous quote goes, "Extraordinary claims require extraor-dinary evidence." If you're telling me that rubbing this cream on my leg is going to reduce my muscle soreness and improve the contractile proper-ties of my muscle, I need to see some proof. A blog post and a YouTube video is not enough. Twitter followers are not credentials. You can't just believe the advice that somebody's giving you just because they've got a lot of followers on Twitter. I would always tell my students: Don't just believe what I'm telling you verbatim. You have to actually do some independent verification and look at this objectively in every case.

If something seems too good to be true, it likely is. And even if you find some data supporting an argument that a supplement, a compres-sion garment, or any other tool works, you must consider not only the source but also who paid for the study, and how that entity might ben-efit from its results.

To begin to find worthwhile evidence whether supplements are worth your time, search in PubMed (pubmed.ncbi.nlm.nih.gov) by the supplement name, and add keywords like *athlete*, *recovery*, and the name of your sport.

MULTIVITAMINS AND MINERALS

If you're eating a varied diet full of plant-based foods and your weight is holding steady, you're receiving adequate amounts of vitamins and minerals and have no need for a daily multivitamin and mineral supple-ment. But if you are limiting your food intake or do not eat certain foods for ethical or personal reasons, a multivitamin may help ensure you get adequate amounts of B vitamins; vitamins C, D, and E; beta carotene; and selenium. Another exception would be mineral supplementation (calcium, iron, magnesium, and zinc) for athletes with a history of anemia, especially those who don't eat red meat. Iron supplementation should happen under the direction of a health care professional because taking too much iron can be very harmful.

ANTIOXIDANTS

A healthy diet including a variety of fruit should give you plenty of anti-oxidants, which help combat damage from free radicals released during exercise. However, supplementation can ensure you're doing what you can to combat inflammation. One recent study showed that increased antioxidant consumption after endurance events can aid in recovery by reducing the damage free radicals do to the muscles.[2]

A varied diet rich in fruits and vegetables with bright colors will give you plenty of dietary antioxidants. If you need to supplement, you can turn to red and purple juices, such as grape juice, tart cherry juice, pomegranate juice, and açai juice. These also make a nice mocktail in combination with club soda. The research on such juices is ongoing, so check the most current results on a medical research database such as PubMed before making your decision to supplement (figure 10.1).

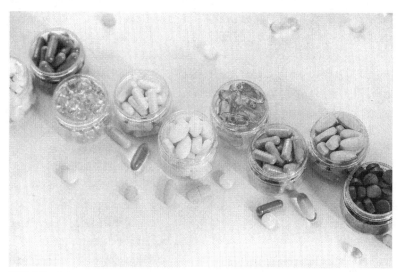

FIGURE 10.1
You should have clear, evidence-based reasons to take any supplement. *Getty Images/Yana Tatevosian*

ESSENTIAL FATTY ACIDS

Essential fatty acids are called "essential" because we must take them in through our diet; our bodies don't generate them on their own. We need both alpha-lineolic acids (ALAs), from omega-3 fats, and lineolic acids, from omega-6 fats. But the typical Western diet contains far too much of the omega-6 fats, which can promote inflammation, in proportion to the omega-3 fats, which can combat inflammation. The best approach is to correct this imbalance by consuming more omega-3 fatty acids from fatty cold-water fish such as salmon, mackerel, sardines, and herring, and from plant sources like flaxseed and walnuts.

A second approach is to supplement with omega-3 intake from fish oil or flaxseed oil. You'll find various fish oil supplements on the market. Look for one that contains both EPA (eicosapentaenoic acid) and DHA (docosahexaenoic acid); these are the omega-3 fats your body needs. Examine the source of the fish oil—is it from cold-water fish like salmon and anchovies? If ethical farming matters to you, you'll want to investigate the farming practices. Is the supplement pure and fresh, and can the producer cite a third-party tester to guarantee these claims? (It seems safest to choose an independently inspected producer.) Is it in capsule form, and if so, what is the source of the capsule? (Vegetarians won't want a gelatin capsule.)

Krill oil, made from small marine creatures, contains EPA and DHA as well as the antioxidant astaxanthin. There is some concern about depletion of Antarctic krill, so if you want to support sustainable farming, do your research on the source of your supplement if you choose krill oil. Those who do use krill oil report there's less of the fishy burping that can be associated with fish oil. You will also find algae-based alternatives appropriate for vegans and vegetarians—another way for everyone to get around the fishiness. This is what I use personally, and omega-3s are the one supplement I take.

Or look for flaxseed or flaxseed oil. Both contain alpha-lineolic acid (ALA), which your body will synthesize into EPA and DHA, at some metabolic cost. (Eating fish or taking fish oil supplements will be a more direct source of EPA and DHA.)

The World Health Organization recommends healthy adults consume 0.3–0.5 grams of EPA and DHA per day, and a larger amount—around a gram—of ALA. Read the label on your fish oil supplement to find how much you'd need to take to reach that range. The more concentrated the better. If you choose flaxseeds instead, you can eat a tablespoon of seeds to receive about a teaspoon's worth of oil. Either contains about 2 grams of ALA.

Storage for omega-3 supplements can be tricky. Because flaxseed oil is highly unsaturated, it should be kept cold and shielded from light, and package contents should be consumed within a few weeks of being opened. If flax oil is heated, it loses its beneficial properties. If a package goes rancid, it can lead to illness, and in some circumstances, it can change into trans fat.

If you are going to use flaxseeds, you'll want to grind them so that they can be processed by your body (instead of leaving your system in the same state they entered, or worse, massing together and clogging up the plumbing entirely). You can grind flaxseeds in a coffee grinder or with a mortar and pestle. Grind seeds as you'll be using them, or grind a whole batch ahead of time and store it in the freezer.

PROTEIN SUPPLEMENTS

Marketers try to convince athletes that they need protein powder to help rebuild muscles during recovery periods between workouts. But the average Westerner is already eating more than the amount of protein required per day. If you are in doubt about whether you are meeting your protein needs, schedule an appointment with a sports nutritionist. For most of us, there's really no need to supplement with protein powders; eating lean protein from healthy sources will suffice and is preferable. But if you eat a vegetarian or vegan diet, you might benefit from paying extra attention to protein intake.

PREPACKAGED RECOVERY SUPPLEMENTS

Postworkout Beverages

We've seen the importance of the recovery snack or meal, especially following longer workouts. Many companies market prepackaged recovery drinks and drink mixes. When you don't have the logistical ability to make your own food, these can come in handy as a postworkout snack. So, however, can any range of non–recovery specific items, from SlimFast and Ensure shakes to premixed yogurt smoothies. Let your palate, your budget, and your experience be your guide.

Recovery Supplements

Beyond the snack, some companies offer capsules to deliver branched-chain amino acids (BCAAs, consisting of leucine, isoleucine, and valine), glucosamine, and other ingredients with the goal of targeting recovery. Studies are inconclusive about their benefits, as you will see later in the chapter. Do your own thorough research in conjunction with your health care team. Again, be sure you are getting quality training, food, and sleep and that you aren't reaching for a bottle to make up for deficiencies in your self-care.

OTHER SUPPLEMENTS

It can be very difficult to separate marketing from reality when researching supplements because producers can make claims about their products that are not clinically proven. According to the American Dietetic Association, only a few supplements marketed as ergogenic aids actually perform as claimed.[3] They include creatine, caffeine, sports drinks/bars/gels, and protein supplements. Nutritionist Scott Tindal explains of creatine: "people are scared of it because they think it's going to make them super bulky and carry extra weight. But for endurance athletes, it really is one of those supplements that has a very positive impact on performance. And if the athlete is a vegan or a vegetarian, then it will have a bigger impact, because creatine is mainly consumed through animal products."

Next I discuss some commonly used supplements that are not specifically proven to work for recovery but that may be worth a try in consultation with your coach and health care provider.

Amino Acids

While protein supplementation is probably unnecessary, there may be benefits to consuming BCAAs before and after your workout. BCAAs have been shown to reduce delayed-onset muscle soreness (DOMS) and to improve immune function.[4] The latter can be a useful benefit: Athletes in heavy training are susceptible to infection because their immune systems are suppressed.

Similarly, supplementing with the amino acid glutamine can boost the immune system, although a diet with adequate protein consumption should give you plenty of glutamine. Athletes with overtraining syndrome exhibit low plasma glutamine levels,[5] but that does not directly imply that supplementing with glutamine will prevent overtraining or enhance recovery.

A supplement protocol for amino acids might include adding 5–10 grams of BCAA powder to your breakfast and your postworkout snack each day, and/or adding 5 grams of glutamine to your postworkout snack.

Ginseng

Another potential immune system booster is ginseng. It can also help the body adapt to stress, which has obvious beneficial applications for your recovery. But its effects on performance and recovery have not been conclusively proven,[6] and it is complicated to secure a quality preparation and then to follow the necessary protocol of cyclical dosing. Focus your attention instead on smart training, adequate rest, and whole-foods nutrition.

PHARMACEUTICAL PRODUCTS

Pharmaceutical products are not supplements and will not aid in your general recovery. If you need to take over-the-counter products to dampen your pain so that you can continue training, consider it a red flag. That's a sign it's time to visit your health care provider to investigate the root of the problem. Perhaps it's an overuse injury that would respond quickly with rest or corrective exercises. Better to get an answer immediately than to attempt to train through a problem that could wind up seriously damaging your body and jettisoning your race schedule.

Many athletes reach for nonsteroidal anti-inflammatory medications such as Advil (ibuprofen) and Aleve (naproxen) when they feel the aches and pains associated with training. If you find your hand on the bottle, stop and ask yourself why you're taking the medication. What hurts? Is the pain relegated to a particular area? If so, when was the onset of the pain? Can you see a reason for the pain: a drastic increase in mileage, a fall, overworn running shoes? It may be time to work with a professional to get to the root of your pain, instead of masking its symptoms.

Taking NSAIDs in large dosages can actually interfere with your body's ability to recover by slowing your healing time. Overuse of NSAIDs can lead to a host of problems, from gastrointestinal trouble to kidney problems, as your doctor will tell you. By blocking the COX enzyme, they increase the likelihood of stomach upset, including nausea, and of diarrhea. And prescription NSAIDs that act as COX-2 inhibitors can increase your risk of heart attack. Speak to your health care professional about any medications and supplements you ingest. Take care before using any over-the-counter medication to mask what your body is experiencing.

Quality Matters

While supplements receive very little oversight, quality producers will meet the FDA's Good Manufacturing Practices (GMPs), and will have their ingredients supported by a certificate of analysis (COA). The U.S. Pharmacopeia (USP) is a third-party nonprofit organization that tests products' purity and strength, as well as their manufacturing standards. Check that your chosen supplement has been approved by the USP or another third-party organization. You can also look for these elements:

- Organic ingredients
- The presence or absence of wheat, corn, or soy (if you are sensitive to them) and of artificial colors or flavorings
- Sustainable farming practices (if you want to consider the ethical implications of your purchase)
- Expiration date (ideally in the future)
- Storage instructions (if the product should be kept in the pantry or refrigerator)

QUICK TIPS

- Be wary of any "miracle cures" and aim to get your nutrients from real food.
- Increasing the amount of omega-3 fatty acids you ingest can aid your recovery.
- Juices rich in antioxidants such as tart cherry juice are also promising for recovery (and tasty).
- NSAIDs are not a recovery aid; in fact, they can interfere with your body's natural recovery process.

Cold and Heat

Time: little

Cost: low

Accessibility: good

Confidence: mixed

Contraindications: avoid heat when muscles are inflamed

Like many recovery techniques, the effective application of cold and heat depends on the individual athlete. Studies have returned conflicting results on the effectiveness of various treatments—the importance of the temperature of the cold or heat applied, the amount of time spent in temperature therapy, and whether there is a difference between dry heat and moist heat's effect on the body—and on the exact processes at play during heat and cold therapy. Some of the most recent research shows that despite the widespread custom of taking ice baths, cold doesn't seem to help much in recovery from endurance or speed training. Worse, it might negatively affect muscular adaptation after resistance training.[1] Another study showed that a placebo of soaking in tepid water delivered better recovery measurements than a cold bath.² Regardless of the spotty and sometimes contradictory research, many athletes report a benefit from using both cold and heat for recovery. Thus you should experiment to find what works best for you. Your personal reaction to and appreciation of these methods will determine whether they enhance the quality of your recovery.

While "Iceman" Wim Hof's ascendance has encouraged people to take cold plunges, the science now argues further against the use of ice baths than it did 10 years ago. Before taking a cold plunge, or emptying your ice tray into your tub, consider why you are contemplating cold water immersion. Is it because your coach—or a social media influencer—suggested it? On what replicable evidence? Is it because you want to feel tough, or alive? Is more discomfort in your day useful, or is it counterproductive? Ice baths can feel like a form of hazing: something coaches endured in their student-athlete days, that they then perpetuate without considering whether the concept is borne out by the evidence.

In general, ice is used to combat the inflammation incurred in training, both generally, from repetitive pounding, and specifically, from acute trauma such as a crash or a tackle. When soft tissues are in an acute stage of damage, adding heat will only aggravate this inflammation. Cooling the tissues, whether through a stay in a cold bath or direct application of an ice pack, will combat excessive inflammation and prevent or minimize edema (swelling). Subsequent removal of the cold stimulus then encourages renewed blood flow to the area, bringing in oxygen and cellular chemicals to speed up recovery while removing the negative byproducts of exercise and inflammation. Ice baths can also have an analgesic effect, repressing the sense of pain associated with inflammation.

Spending time in a warm environment, however—either a dry one such as a sauna or a wet one such as a steam room or a whirlpool—can increase circulation and loosen stiff muscles. A warm room or bath can feel nurturing, too, encouraging relaxation and enabling the parasympathetic nervous system to facilitate recovery.

COLD

Cold is used to counter inflammation, to encourage vasoconstriction (tightening in the blood vessels), and to numb pain. This has its place in recovery from the general trauma of training, as well as in recovery from a specific injury. If you have an injury that requires icing, check back in your training history to consider where you might be overdoing it and give recovery extra focus.

Ice Bath

Many athletes swear by the postworkout ice bath, which they theorize helps reduce inflammation and move waste products from the muscles. But studies do not bear out this effect with evidence; a placebo of a neutral temperature bath did better on recovery measurements than cold water did.[3]

Cool, not freezing cold water seems to have an analgesic effect, reducing pain if not directly affecting recovery.[4] If you live near the ocean, a quiet river, or a stream, you may have a natural cool bath handy. Many triathletes revisit the body of water they raced in after the event to help cool down the body's core temperature. Taking a cool bath to reduce inflammation and hasten recovery builds on this practice. Ultrarunner Charlie Engle remembers, "In Monterey, California, our long run started and finished in Carmel Beach at the bottom of Ocean Avenue. At the end of every run, I walked into the water up to my waist and stood for 5 minutes. That's cold water, in the mid-50s, more than cold enough. There's a spiritual aspect, thanks for the gift of the day." If you have access to an outdoor pool in the off-season, you can submerge your legs up to your hips for the cool-bath effect.

If cool water immersion makes you happy—and better yet, if it gives you time to socialize with training partners or fellow competitors and to process your experience, or to give thanks and appreciation for your strong body—it's probably a net gain to do it. Just keep clear eyes about whether and how it helps, as the scientific mechanisms are still unclear.

•

Direct Application of Ice

Ice is a common treatment to reduce inflammation associated with the acute phase of an injury. The standard protocol is to apply ice for 10 to 15 minutes, and sometimes to repeat applications after 20 minutes off, up to three times a day. Longer application of ice can begin to freeze the tissues—effectively creating frostbite.

Coach Peter Magill prefers local application of ice to an ice bath, arguing that the ice bath can interfere with the necessary inflammatory response. If you finish a run and have even minor soreness that feels out of the ordinary, he advises, "get ice on it right away, within about 15 minutes before your body has a chance to react to the irritation by creating more inflammation. While you can't have recovery without minor inflammation, it's a snowball effect to major inflammation." Minor inflammation is part of the natural healing process, but major inflammation can equate to major soreness and pain and can indicate a serious injury requiring medical attention.

If you find yourself with soreness that needs ice or with an incipient injury, check your training log for signs of too much intensity. You may need to adjust your training to alleviate stress on your body. If you do choose to ice, here are some ways to make a comfortable cold pack:

1. Freeze a paper cup full of water. Rub your sore spots with the ice, effectively giving yourself an ice massage. As the ice melts, peel the paper back. Since the ice is constantly moving, the risk of damaging your skin is low, but be careful.

2. Use frozen vegetables (small peas work well) or frozen rice in a bag. They will conform around most joints. Lay a thin towel between the bag and your skin for protection from frostbite.

3. Create a slurry of one part rubbing alcohol to three parts water in a zippable plastic bag. (You can experiment with the ratio, depending on freezer temperature and your preference for the viscosity of the ice.) The alcohol lowers the solution's freezing point so that it stays liquid in the freezer. This pack is especially good for wrapping

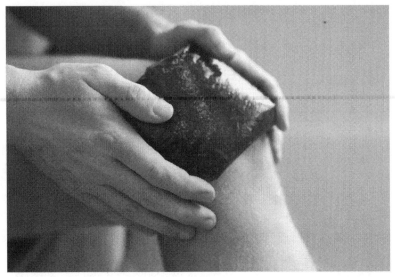

FIGURE 11.1
Be aware of how frequently you feel like ice is necessary—too much icing could be a sign of too much training load. *Getty Images/AndreyPopov*

knobby areas such as knees or ankles (figure 11.1). Because the solution will not warm up as quickly as vegetables, you will need to be careful to protect your skin from frostbite.

Cryotherapy Chambers

Beyond the ice bath is a cold-freeze (cryotherapy) chamber, which you might find in training facilities and recovery studios. While these might be interesting for the stories, they don't seem to show much benefit,[5] and they can be quite intense. Your time and money may be better spent on high-quality food and a cozy pair of pajamas (call them "recovery garments" if you like) that you can wear to relax in.

HEAT

Many cultures have long used heated rooms and baths for therapeutic treatment—think of Roman baths, Finnish saunas, and Japanese bathhouses. In a heated environment, blood flow to the skin is increased, along with perspiration. Beyond the physiological benefits of heated rooms, a short stay in a warm environment can feel nurturing and relaxing, increasing parasympathetic nervous function and thus hastening recovery.

Sauna

Spending time in the sauna has been shown to reduce blood pressure in hypertensive subjects and to help those with respiratory diseases. Better yet, recent studies show that a postworkout trip to the sauna may improve blood volume, overall cardiovascular health, VO2 max, and speed at lactate threshold.[6]

Depending on the facility you use, the sauna may be at 180 degrees Fahrenheit or even hotter. Take care to monitor your response, and move out of the sauna for breaks whenever you feel you want them. Aim to stay 15–30 minutes a few days a week, ideally directly after your workout. More is not necessarily better, especially if you do not find the sauna relaxing.

A traditional (Finnish) sauna is between 80 and 100 degrees Celsius, or 160–210 degrees Fahrenheit. Newer infrared saunas operate at lower temperatures but use far-infrared light to generate heat within the subjects' bodies. One study showed infrared saunas improved neuromuscular recovery after endurance training over use of a traditional sauna.[7]

Both infrared and traditional saunas are widely available at gyms, spas, and recovery studios (figure 11.2). You may also want to buy your own for home use—a small infrared sauna will set you back a few thousand dollars, and backyard barrel saunas cost around USD$5,000 or more, so try using one at a gym, spa, or studio before you splurge. And remember: attention to the fundamentals will get you far more bang for your buck than dropping several grand on a fancy toy.

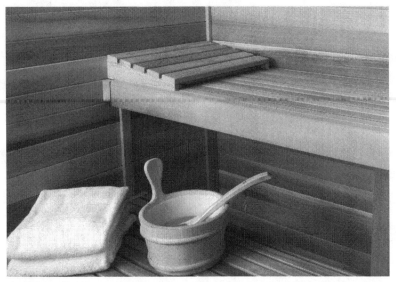

FIGURE 11.2
Recent evidence shows that sauna visits can enhance your workout gains. *Getty Images/Sportstock*

Steam Room

The steam room is often heated to 112 degrees, with very high humidity. Those with respiratory conditions such as asthma may respond well to the humidity; others may find the steam room oppressive. While the temperature in a steam room is lower than that in a sauna, it is sufficient to begin increasing core temperature. Stay for only brief periods, no more than 20 minutes.

Whirlpool

A whirlpool, or hot tub, combines warm temperatures with the benefits of water therapy. The hydrostatic pressure of water is beneficial for reducing swelling, and the movement of water over the body will relax both muscles and mind while increasing circulation. Take care, however, not to add heat to already inflamed tissue, as heat will only feed the inflammation, slowing your recovery time.

Warm Bath

Some athletes prefer the warm bath to the ice bath. Matt Dixon says, "I am not a fan of ice at all (except for specific injuries), as it leads to tightening of the muscles. Post-workouts, many take ice baths to prevent swelling. I find the negatives often override the positives, with tight muscles following. I prefer a warm bath."

A warm bath—cooler than the 100-plus-degree water of a whirlpool—can be relaxing and is easily created at home. Ultrarunner Keith Straw says, "I love a nice hot bath while drinking a nice cold beer! Complete relaxation—the hot bath and the cold, bubbly beer. None of that painful stuff!" Coach Greg McMillan jokes, "That's what New Zealanders call icing from the inside."

Direct Application of Heat

A heating pad or warm pack can be a comfort for sore muscles, especially in the back, neck, and shoulders. Before applying such heat, consider the cause of the soreness. If your muscles have been overworked and may be inflamed, adding heat may only exacerbate the situation, compounding your soreness and slowing your recovery. If you're feeling stiff or would like to warm up the muscles before a massage, whether self-massage, professional massage, or massage performed by a friend, some heat may help set the stage for better release.

There are two types of heat that can be used to warm the muscles. Most heating pads, despite what their labels may claim, provide dry heat. Heating pads are easy to use and convenient for warming the back. It's difficult, though, to make a heating pad conform to certain areas of the body, including the neck and shoulders. Here, a gel pack or a steamed towel is more useful. They provide moist heat, which many people prefer. As with other modalities, determine what works best for you. Be sure that the temperature is not too hot, and stop use after 20 minutes. You may need a towel to act as a buffer between your skin and the heat source. Pay close attention to the sensation to ensure that it remains safely pleasant.

ALTERNATING COLD AND HEAT

Contrast therapy (alternating between heat and cold) is a common recovery technique, with athletes spending a few minutes in cold, moving to heat, returning to cold, and repeating for a few rounds, usually finishing with cold. It produces an appreciable response in the body because athletes can feel vasoconstriction and vasodilation—the pumping of the blood vessels, which constrict and dilate—as they move from cold to hot and back again.

Some studies suggest that contrast therapy might counteract recovery. For example, a 1989 study of Finnish swimmers showed that alternating heat and cold reduces plasma volume (that is, leads to dehydration) and elevates stress hormones in the body.[8] This is the opposite of what we're searching for with recovery. But the practice is still popular, and as with separate applications of cold and heat, anecdotal evidence shows that contrast therapy can be very effective. If you enjoy alternating heat and cold, you should schedule such contrast therapy after a workout and keep it separate from your key workouts. If you take care to stay hydrated, you might find contrast therapy beneficial.

INFLAMMATION IS NOT THE ENEMY

Training involves imposing a stress on the body so that it will grow back stronger. Inflammation is a natural by-product of this imposition of stress, and the reaction inflammation instigates in the body begins the recovery process. Thus inflammation is not the enemy; it is even to be desired.

The problem occurs when inflammation outstrips what the body can handle during the recovery window. Thus the goal of ice, or alternating ice and heat, or any of the anti-inflammatory recovery modalities described in this book, is to combat *excess* inflammation that becomes a precursor to injury in a specific location or illness in the entire system.

QUICK TIPS

- Use cold to combat inflammation caused by training.

- Heat can loosen stiff muscles and increase circulation but can also aggravate existing inflammation.

- After long or hard workouts, aim to spend 10 to 15 minutes in an ice bath of 50 to 60 degrees.

- Eating a warm snack in the ice bath will make it more comfortable and will hasten your recovery.

- A frozen slurry of rubbing alcohol and water in a 1 to 3 ratio, mixed in a sealable bag, makes a handy ice pack that conforms to knobby body parts.

- When directly applying heat or ice, use a towel as a buffer to protect your skin from frostbite.

12

Home Technological Aids

Athletes are always looking for the next tool to improve their performance. While getting quality sleep, reducing stress, and improving nutrition hold the key to recovery and success as an athlete, it's tempting to drop a few dollars on tools that promise to give you an edge on the competition. And when your social media feed and news reader are full of posts recommending certain tools—often with an affiliate link, to earn revenue for the mention—it can be tough to know where your money is best spent. If you haven't upgraded your mattress, consulted with a sports nutritionist, and worked with a sports psychiatrist to strategize for your season and maximize the ways you handle stress, spend your money there first! In this chapter, we'll look at compression garments and other easily accessible products that are used externally to enhance recovery.

COMPRESSION SOCKS

Time: little

Cost: low

Accessibility: good

Confidence: high

Contraindications: improperly sized garments

What Compression Socks Do

Compression socks, tight knee-high socks made of compressive fabrics, are designed to improve venous return by enhancing the natural pump action of the calf muscles (figure 12.1). Many companies manufacture socks for use during exercise as well as socks for use during recovery. They can differ in the location of compression and in the materials used.

Compression garments for the lower leg come in two styles: full socks and calf sleeves, which leave the feet uncovered. Those aren't ideal for recovery, as they can trap fluids in the feet. Graduated-compression socks are tighter in the ankles than the calves. For running, sleeves work fine, since the action of running will recirculate fluids. But beware running in the sleeves if they hit right at your ankle. When ultrarunner Charlie Engle had tendonitis in his ankle, he found the sleeves hit at just the wrong point for his running stride. He said, "I put on compression sleeves, and where that thing stopped, it compressed. The tendon moving through the sheath, as it became swollen inside, made things worse; it exacerbated the situation."

The material in compression garments can be uniformly compressive or graduated, so that the pressure is firmer at the bottom and lighter at the top. These are the socks generally used by athletes. The degree of compression also varies in the socks. Over-the-counter socks from the drugstore will apply 10–20 mmHg of pressure; medical-grade prescription socks will go to 50 mmHg or higher. Most socks marketed to athletes fall somewhere in between. For graduated socks, a pressure of more than 18 mmHg at the foot, decreasing toward the calf, is needed to improve venous return. More can work, but if there is too much pressure, it can begin to impair blood flow—working counter to its intended use.[1] The amount of compression you receive will depend not only on the product you choose but also on the way it fits. A sock that's a little too big will offer less pressure.

While studies have focused on subjects wearing compression socks for many hours at a stretch, this isn't feasible for the average athlete, nor would it be comfortable, especially in warmer weather. Instead, if you are going to try compression socks, aim to wear them for a few hours in the afternoon or evening following a hard workout. And if you are traveling, wear the socks but bring another pair of regular, noncompression socks in case they grow uncomfortable.

Data on how long to wear the socks are inconclusive. One rule of thumb: Wear your socks for twice as long as the workout you're recovering from. Thus a 90-minute run could be followed by a three-hour stint in socks, and you might sleep in your recovery socks or tights following a four- or five-hour ride.

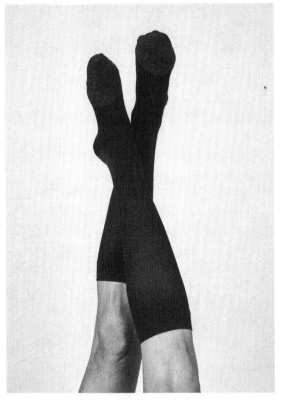

FIGURE 12.1
Compression socks, just like legs up the wall pose, help return fluids from your lower legs for processing. *Getty Images/nito100*

Expect your compression garments to maintain their compression for about six months, depending on how often you wear and wash them. In time, they will loosen. Some experts suggest 50 washes as a reasonable amount of wear to expect, while others suggest having a pair for training, a pair for racing, and a pair for recovery and replacing them all once a year.

Finally, some products combine compression and ice. Dave Strassburg, creator of the Strassburg Sock used to treat plantar fasciitis, offers a sleeve that contains pockets for ice. Sold under the Runner's Remedy label, there are models targeting the Achilles tendon, the arch of the foot, and the shins. If you find you have to ice specific areas in your body regularly, or if your pain becomes localized to a specific joint or even to only one side of your body, it's time to look further into the root of the issue by investigating your training load, your attention to recovery, and your biomechanics.

How Effective Compression Socks Are

How effective are compression socks for recovery? This question really has two parts. First, does wearing compression socks *during* exercise affect recovery afterward? And second, does wearing compression socks *after* exercise affect recovery?

Regarding the first question, the answer is probably. A New Zealand study of runners wearing knee-high graduated compression socks while running both a shuttle run (back-and-forth agility sprints) and a 10K found that the group wearing the socks reported significantly less delayed-onset muscle soreness than the control group, who did not wear the socks.[2] This has interesting implications for recovery: An athlete experiencing less muscle soreness after the run should be ready for another run sooner.

Another study points to the same conclusion. A study testing the effect of compression socks on maximal exercise performance and lactate recovery rate after exercise found the socks to have no effect on performance. But the subjects wearing compression socks exhibited a faster lactate recovery rate after exercise.[3] Of course, thinking on lactic acid has changed in recent years, and it is now thought not to have an effect on postexercise soreness. It will leave the bloodstream on its own shortly after a workout—even after a high-intensity workout, blood lactate is back to resting levels within 90 minutes. Thus, blood lactate levels may not be important.

The second question is whether wearing recovery socks *after* a workout will enhance recovery. On this subject, a few studies have been conducted. One study on netball and basketball players measured the effects of wearing compression tights for 48 hours after plyometric exercises. They found an insignificant effect on performance for the control group. Interestingly, the group wearing the tights reported less pain, and many of the subjects adopted regular use of compression gear as part of their training.[4] A randomized controlled trial of athletes who wore socks for two days after running a marathon showed a functional recovery benefit to the compression socks over placebo. They were able to perform better on a treadmill test two weeks postrace.[5]

Anecdotal evidence certainly supports the use of compression socks for recovery. Many elite athletes swear by them. Runner Nate Jenkins says that while he's tried the socks in workouts and hasn't noticed any difference in performance, they work well for recovery. "I put them on right away, while the snack's in the blender," he says. "I'll keep them on for two to four hours." Ultrarunner Jamie Donaldson says: "I always wear compression socks during an ultra and after. I feel that they increase circulation from my legs back to my heart. I never have swelling and have minimal soreness."

Physiologist Stephen McGregor says that while some of the marketing for compression socks is simply that—marketing—they are useful for those who can't get off their feet after workouts. "If you have a life and have to walk around," he says, "compression clothing will help return the blood for processing."

The socks are also useful for travel. U.S. Olympic bronze medalist Shalane Flanagan says, "Whenever I fly internationally, I use compression socks. It helps my legs." Many of the athletes I talked to echoed

Flanagan. I wear the socks myself during winter travel, when I can hide them under pants; in the summer they are too warm.

The bottom line: if you enjoy wearing the socks, do. They are useful for recovery. Reconsider, however, whether they are worth wearing in a race. In a triathlon, the amount of time it takes to don them might not be worth any potential speed gained by wearing them.

CREAMS

> **Time:** little
>
> **Cost:** low
>
> **Accessibility:** good
>
> **Confidence:** high
>
> **Contraindications:** allergy; contamination is possible; wintergreen oil can be fatal in overdoses

Bengay, Icy-Hot, Biofreeze, Prossage, and Chinese White Flour are all examples of creams and liniments that athletes apply to muscles. Usually, they are used for minor aches and pains and therefore intended to be more therapeutic than used purely for recovery. Their effect is usually to confuse the nerve endings and draw attention away from the original issue and toward the skin. Many of these products contain wintergreen oil, so take caution in applying them. The oil's active ingredient, methyl salicylate, carries anti-inflammatory properties and can be fatal in very high doses.

Massaging such creams into the skin can be pleasant, as any massage can be. You might have an equally or more pleasant experience massaging scented lotion into your skin, without any of the tingling or burning associated with medicated lotions. Lavender lotion smells nice, for example, and aromatherapy practitioners say the scent of lavender is relaxing.

Arnica is a homeopathic remedy available at natural-foods stores in both cream and gel format. A few randomized, double-blind studies suggest that arnica speeds healing from bruises and minor swelling, while other studies point to a placebo effect. Application of arnica for minor aches isn't going to hurt you, but any pain that goes beyond slight muscle soreness or is specific to one side or area of your body is a sign to back off your training and to consider consulting a medical professional. Similarly, if you have pain that prompts you to repeatedly apply Bengay or other topical balms, you should visit a medical professional to have the cause of the injury diagnosed.

CBD creams show promise in pain management for diseased people. Their use in athletes as a recovery aid hasn't been studied much.[6] CBD products may ultimately help with sleep—and thus directly enhance one of your most powerful recovery tools. For now, if you find it helpful, it shouldn't hurt, but you'll find a wide range of products, strengths, and manufacturing practices.

This brings us to a final word of caution: As with supplements, you must be very careful about applying products to your body. Many are not subject to government regulation and may contain substances on the World Anti-Doping Agency (WADA) banned list. If you are subject to drug testing—or simply concerned about your well-being—be careful with every product, whether you ingest it or use it topically.

EPSOM SALTS

Time: little

Cost: low

Accessibility: good

Confidence: high—as a placebo

Contraindications: none

When it comes to Epsom salt (magnesium sulfate) baths, it seems to be the bath itself—not the salts—that has the effect. The hydrostatic pressure of the water on your body helps reduce swelling, and the feeling of floating in a bath can be heightened, if only incrementally, by the addition of salt. A warm bath is relaxing, and adding Epsom salts or a pricier, scented version of bath salts will enhance the experience. The ritual of drawing and soaking in a warm bath, possibly with low lighting, candles, and soft music, is relaxing and restorative in ways beyond the arguable benefits of adding Epsom salts.

Magnesium sulfate is said to have anti-inflammatory properties, though simply soaking in it would be an indirect way to receive those benefits, and absorption and metabolization would depend on the athlete. Some magnesium from the Epsom salts is absorbed through the skin. A 2006 study by Dr. Rosemary Waring showed that magnesium sulfate levels increased in subjects who took hot baths with Epsom salts for 12 minutes at a time. But the study was small and funded by the magnesium sulfate industry. It has since been both touted on the internet and roundly discredited.[7]

The bottom line is that soaking in Epsom salts, a cup or two to a bath, won't hurt you. If you buy the generic salts at your drugstore, it won't affect your wallet much, either; they cost only a few dollars per gallon. If you enjoy the scent of a blended bath salt, you can splurge on a commercial product or mix your own salts by adding dried lavender or rosebuds, available at most natural-foods stores, to Epsom salts.

QUICK TIPS

- Look for graduated compression garments, such as socks that are tighter at the ankle and looser through the calf.
- Replace your recovery compression garments somewhere between 50 washings and 12 months of use.
- If you have aches that keep you reaching for topical creams like Bengay, arnica, or CBD creams, be sure you have the right biomechanics and work/rest ratio.
- While Epsom salts' effect on recovery is dubious, it's relaxing to take a warm bath.

13

Other Technological Aids

Time: moderate
Cost: moderate to expensive
Accessibility: low to moderate
Confidence: moderate
Contraindications: using technological aids to mask injury

In contrast to the home-use items described in chapter 12, other devices are used mainly in clinical settings or in studios where shared use defrays the cost. In the decade since the first edition of this book, not only have gyms added "recovery stations" with accessories for foam rolling but also entire recovery studios have opened. These offer everything from assisted stretching to oxygen chambers, automated massage devices like the Normatec (which was just becoming mainstream a decade ago), and sensory deprivation / float tanks. What might be worth seeking out and spending money on? Once you're sure you've maximized your sleep, nutrition, and stress management, it's a question of time, budget, and access.

ULTRASOUND

For team sports athletes with access to athletic trainers, ultrasound and electrostimulation are primarily used in rehabilitating after injury, although some athletes use them for general recovery. Studies are inconclusive about the benefits of ultrasound for therapeutic use in recovering from sports injuries. A 2010 study concluded that receiving real ultrasound versus sham ultrasound made no difference in recovery from an ankle injury.[1] A 2004 study showed that ultrasound does not speed muscle recovery after a contusion.[2] Indeed, it might lead an athlete into returning to workouts too soon, because muscles feel better following ultrasound treatments. Apart from crashes and falls, endurance athletes don't suffer contusions during training, but the study argues against the use of ultrasound for simple muscle recovery. Still, some athletes enjoy the ultrasound machine. If you find yourself turning to it often, you should consider whether you are developing an overuse injury. Examine your training log for signs of overdoing it.

ELECTROSTIMULATION

E-stim devices such as the Globus and the Compex consist of a central unit and wires that hook to electrodes. The athlete places these electrodes on muscle groups, and then the unit sends electrical stimulation into the nerves, forcing the muscles to contract. (E-stim works on muscles, while TENS units, which look similar, are designed to stimulate nerves.) Essentially, it's a passive form of active recovery. The "active recovery" programs on the units purport to release endorphins, relax the muscles, and increase blood flow, thus eliminating toxins faster. (Note: as you'll read in chapter 14, on massage, *toxins* is a catch-all word, and many things we consider "toxins" are part of the natural process of exertion and recovery.)

One study tested electrical stimulation as a recovery modality for endurance athletes and found that, because it "improve[s] blood return to the heart," it makes a good modality to "enhance recovery and restore muscle working capacity."[3] Likewise, Italian researchers found that futsal players (futsal is a variant on indoor soccer) who received electrostimulation as a recovery modality reported a significantly greater perception of recovery benefit than those who did not, suggesting that their enthusiasm for the next game would be greater.[4] This psychological effect is not to be discounted. Finally, many elite athletes testify to the effect of electrical muscle stimulation, although some athletes report finding the devices difficult to manage. I enjoyed testing the Globus machine, and my children thrilled to the sight of my quadriceps twitching during its Active Recovery mode, but I must admit I noticed little difference in the quality of my muscular recovery. The machines might serve a therapeutic benefit, but for healthy athletes who could go for a 20-minute swim, spin, or walk, actual movement would trump having a machine activate your muscles. Still, the time I took to rest still on the couch and emphasize my recovery between workouts was well spent, regardless of whether the Globus unit effected any change.

The bottom line is these devices have a lot of marketing behind them and not as much science. Remember, time, sleeping well, and eating right are the most important recovery tools. If you have the money to afford an e-stim unit and the time to sit with the electrodes in place, go for it. But be sure you are first getting enough rest and healthy food and that you are training wisely.

FLOAT TANKS

Float tanks offer the user a period of time in a tank of very salty, shallow body-temperature water, with or without the lid closed to make it dark. When the lid is closed, the tank is a form of sensory deprivation chamber, with very minimal light, little to no sound beyond the sound of your pulse and your breath, and no hard contact between your body and a solid object. If this sounds appealing rather than frightening, and you can find a tank locally that rents by the session, try it out.

Studies are promising about time spent floating leading to positive results in a variety of health issues. Do they work for athletic recovery? It's unclear but not harmful, as a 2019 study on the tanks showed.[5] While Matt Driller, one of the study's authors, says that further research is needed, he finds them promising: "The thing I like the most about float tanks is that they are one of the few times that an athlete is actually forced to be away from their phone and technology and really switch off!" They may also improve sleep, he says (and is studying). But they may not be available to you locally, or if you are traveling to compete, so their use is limited.

OTHER EMERGING TECHNOLOGIES

Depending on where you live and what's hot in the moment, you might find options to lie in an infrared light bed (like a tanning bed but with infrared light), which uses photobiomodulation in an attempt to regenerate tissues faster.[6] Or you might be able to book time in a halotherapy room, breathing air that has been infused with salt. (This shows some promise for respiratory treatments, but not for athletic recovery.)[7]

If you have the budget and time for these, knock yourself out. They shouldn't hurt and, depending on the technology and wavelength, might help cosmetically by stimulating collagen production in your skin, or by giving you a time in the salt cave away from screens and other stressors. But your time is probably spent just as well napping, or prepping a healthy meal. Remember: the fundamentals of sleep, nutrition, and overall stress reduction matter far more than any buzzy new technology. Don't major in the minors, constantly chasing some secret tool. The secret is in the basics.

QUICK TIPS

- Scientific proof of the efficacy of ultrasound and electro-stimulation is scant. Prioritize smart training, good nutrition, and adequate rest over expensive technological aids.
- If you have areas that require ultrasound, be sure you do not have an incipient or existing overuse injury.
- Before spending money on expensive sessions out of the house, check that your sleep, nutrition, and overall stress management strategies are going well.

14

Massage

Time: low to moderate

Cost: moderate to expensive

Accessibility: good in populated areas

Confidence: high

Contraindications: using massage to treat injury

Massage is a popular therapy for athletes and one of the modalities that first springs to mind when you consider recovery. But how, exactly, does it work? What is the right kind of massage to get? When is the right time for a massage? How can you find the best therapist for you? And can we quantify the difference massage makes toward your recovery? In this chapter, I'll answer these questions and more.

THE PHYSIOLOGICAL BENEFITS OF MASSAGE

Does massage work for recovery? If you've ever had a massage, you'll probably answer yes. Many of the benefits of massage are unquantifiable but directly related to your recovery. Massage gives you time away from training, work, family demands, and the screens that tether you to training, work, and family. It helps you reach a state of deep relaxation, and in this way it carries some of the benefits of meditation: lowered blood pressure, emotional stability, a sense of holistic well-being.

Massage has a positive effect on the parasympathetic nervous system, and thereby enhances recovery.[1] When your parasympathetic nervous system is dominant, you have a better sense of relaxation and well-being, and your body is in an optimal state for recovery. This is why meditation, yoga, and general downtime all help, too.

Scientific research reaches various conclusions about massage's effectiveness.[2] A study on NCAA Division I basketball and volleyball players showed that massage was effective in reduction of delayed-onset muscle soreness (DOMS).[3] Subjects were able to perform better on the vertical jump and agility tests after massage to alleviate their soreness. But as another study points out, this could be a negative, because the effects of DOMS linger even after muscle soreness has faded.[4] An athlete might be tempted to return to intense training too soon and wind up injured. A comprehensive 2008 review included the studies testing whether massage is useful for muscle recovery after exercise.[5] It says that while there are many variables that have not been measured—the technique and intensity of the touch, for example—randomized controlled trials do point to massage aiding in recovery. Because the research studies don't prescribe an ideal timing or frequency of massage (figure 14.1), you'll need to work from your own experience.

Effect on Circulation

Scientific studies have found differing effects of massage on circulation. A study conducted at Queen's University in Kingston, Ontario, showed that massage actually decreased the blood flow to the muscles.[6] In that study, subjects who received massage after exercise showed less blood circulation than those who simply rested (passive recovery) and those who practiced active recovery.

But massage therapists argue that massage aids in circulation, and older studies support them. Massage therapist Leah Kangas, who does a

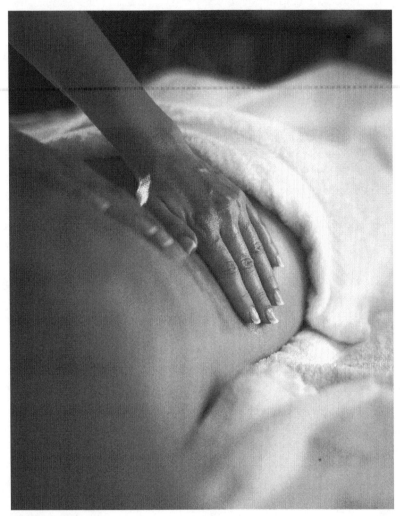

FIGURE 14.1
Look for massage therapists who are familiar with athletes' bodies and needs.
Getty Images/skynesher

lot of work with runners, explains, "Blood carries nutrients throughout the body to heal and repair, and carries away waste products. Massage can help speed up this process by increasing circulation to given muscles or tendons." Massage can also help with movement of lymph through the body; the manual work toward recirculation of blood and lymph may speed recovery. Think of the long strokes from the distal parts of your body—your feet and calves, for example—toward the center.

Older thinking blamed lactic acid produced during exercise for postexercise soreness. Under that paradigm, massage helped remove the lactic acid from the muscles. Newer research shows that lactic acid leaves the muscles fairly quickly after exercise, so it's not the villain it has been painted to be. In fact, Wiltshire's study shows that massage actually slowed the clearance of lactic acid from the muscles after exercise, by reducing circulation. When you hear the phrase "flushing toxins" in conjunction with massage, think less about moving out any residual waste products and more about bringing in the reparative cells that will aid in your adaptation and recovery. Toxins are a bugaboo. Many therapists use the term to describe the natural waste products in the body, often with an admonishment to "drink plenty of water to flush the toxins." Drinking water is generally good advice, especially for athletes, so take that part and ignore the rest.

Exactly what massage does is still unclear. Pat Archer, an athletic trainer and massage therapist and the author of *Therapeutic Massage in Athletics*,[7] explains that massage works, though she admits the precise reasons aren't clear. "It's effective," she says. "We know it helps. We just don't know exactly the full mechanism. They seem to be related to reducing muscle tension and managing the inflammatory process related to microtrauma created by the activity—it's not about circulation, and it's not about lactic acid. It *is* about reducing tension in the muscles after exercise." Archer suggests using specific lymphatic facilitation techniques, strokes with pressure designed to drain the lymphatic system, in conjunction with massage to reduce athletes' recovery time.

Removal of Adhesions

Regular massage can alleviate trigger points and reduce cramping and spasm in the muscles. It can also help with the placement of collagen, preventing adhesions that can cause problems in the muscle and allowing for fuller lengthening and contraction in the fibers.

Adhesions form in the connective tissue, including the fascia, as a result of both tissue breakdown in training and injury, where they set as scar tissue. Kangas uses the orange as an illustration for the fascia and muscle in the human body. "Each muscle fiber has its own little fascial casing, just like the tiny little pulp sections of an orange. Then just like the orange is sectioned, individual muscles are sectioned in the same way. And finally just how an orange is all cased together in the thicker, white section under the peel, so are all of our muscles and organs. Adhesions are when some of these fascial layers get stuck to each other, or adhered." In the case of an acute injury, adhesions are a positive thing, as they provide some structural integrity around the injury site. But scar tissue that doesn't behave like muscle tissue can become problematic, hampering range of motion. Massage helps the scar tissue work more like the muscles or tendons it is repairing.

Ben Benjamin, a sports massage specialist, concurs. "If you're healing and you're moving at the same time, your body heals in the presence of a full range of motion," he explains. Massage can help by encouraging scar tissue to form in appropriate patterns and then to disappear when it is no longer needed for structural support.

Personal Attention

An experienced massage therapist will be able to address your specific issues in ways you won't be able to do alone, which allows for a more targeted approach to your own physiological needs. Carolyn Levy, a massage therapist who worked with the U.S. track team and many players at the University of North Carolina, says her work is more direct than self-massage: "I'm very aware of how I need to approach the tissue, the level of pressure needed. We can get lazy when we do it ourselves. You can't get in specific places." While self-massage is useful—see chapter 15—it can sometimes be too broad a brush. The roller and other self-massage implements can't trace the muscle fibers in the same way the hands of a skilled massage therapist can.

With regular visits, your massage therapist will get to know your body and can let you know when things are changing. If a muscle feels particularly tense or taxed, it may be a sign of incipient injury. Listen to your therapist. Bernard Condevaux, who worked as a *soigneur* (massage therapist, among other things) for USA Cycling, says your massage therapist can be a useful source of outside feedback. "They can tell you things you're denying to yourself," he explains—things like the development of an overuse injury.

Two-time Hawaii Ironman winner Tim DeBoom swears by the power of consistent massage:

> In 1994, I was hit by a car and broke my back. During my rehab I started working with a massage therapist / physical therapist who basically brought me back from the dead. I have now been working with the same therapist for 16 years. She is a vital part of my recovery from training and racing. I go one to two times a week for a pretty deep tissue massage. I also go in for spot work whenever I have any little niggles. Being religious in getting work on my body and the consistency of using the same therapist has kept me from any real debilitating injuries.

Before his win in Kona in 2001, DeBoom got the go-ahead from his massage therapist, who observed that he was "ready to win." And indeed he did. Such observations can instill that extra drop of self-confidence needed for a breakthrough performance—they're an example of not only the physiological benefits of massage but also the psychological benefits.

THE PSYCHOLOGICAL BENEFITS OF MASSAGE

Relaxation

A group of British researchers studied the effect of massage on boxers' recovery between workouts.[8] The fighters who received massage reported a significantly higher perception of recovery, even though the physical testing did not back them up. Regardless of any direct physical link, this perception of recovery is important. Massage confers feelings of relaxation and well-being, which has a direct, positive effect on athletes' perceived recovery.

You'll almost assuredly feel better after any massage, and perception is a big part of recovery. Reducing both muscular and mental tension will certainly help your recovery and your training. Taking time out to focus on your body, to focus on your breath, and to do something that can directly enhance your recovery is well worth the money. In fact, you may achieve deeper relaxation *because* you're paying for it. The massage table is a great place to really let go, away from your smartphone and computer screen, away from the demands of work and family. It echoes training in this way because it allows you a space apart, even as it requires no effort from you at all.

Massage as Therapy

The relationship between massage therapist and athlete can be a positive, supportive one that nurtures the athlete. This happens both through compassionate touch and through the conversation between an athlete and his or her bodyworker—evidence DeBoom's experience. Personally, during heavy training I would spend a good half hour talking to my massage therapist, Pat Kosdan, at our monthly visits before I even climbed on the table. She would ask me what's going on in my body, which usually becomes a conversation about what's going on in my life. When I'm spending more time writing, my body has different issues than when I am deep in a focused training cycle. When I'm stressed with other work or have been teaching yoga intensives, I have different needs. I truly think of Pat as my therapist, with no need to qualify her as my "massage" therapist, and she is a valued adviser.

This interpersonal relationship is important in cycling, where there is a long tradition of traveling with a *soigneur* for support. Condevaux traveled to Beijing in just this role for the 2008 Summer Olympics. He recounts counseling a female mountain biker who needed someone to talk to about her frustrations when her husband wasn't allowed access to the Olympic Village. "When someone's on the table, they'll talk a lot. [Not having her husband around] threw her off. Yes, we did massage, but so much was working her through the issue." On the table, Condevaux says, athletes "can clear their chests and know it stops there."

Ultimately, the number of professional athletes who routinely use and frequently even travel with massage therapists speaks to the importance of massage in training and recovery. Elite running coach Greg McMillan says, "If I had unlimited money, I'd hire a masseuse to be with us all the time. People who are well paid have a masseuse who stretches them out before and after every run. Deena Kastor was really smart, because she married her massage therapist!"

TYPES OF MASSAGE

The two main types of massage therapy offered in the United States are Swedish massage and deep tissue massage. These terms can overlap, naturally. Other, complementary approaches to bodywork include myofascial release, Structural Integration, assisted stretching, and Eastern modalities such as acupuncture, acupressure, and Reiki.

Swedish

Swedish massage generally uses lighter pressure than deep tissue massage. The primary actions in Swedish massage are long, gliding strokes; kneading; tapping; cross-fiber motions; and gentle rocking of the limbs. The strokes generally work from the body's outer edges in toward the heart, following the path of blood flow.

Because Swedish massage is less intense than very deep tissue work, it's acceptable through most, if not all, of the training cycle. Massage therapist Kangas explains, "It's easy to receive a lot of [Swedish massage] while in intense training, and even leading up to and immediately following hard efforts or events, if someone's been receiving the work already."

Deep Tissue

Deep tissue massage works the deeper tissues of the muscles and their interface with fascia, the connective tissue binding the body in every direction. (Remember the orange analogy I used earlier.) The pressure of deep tissue massage will vary not only based on the therapist's approach but also on the needs of the athlete receiving the massage.

Deep tissue work can be uncomfortable to receive, and it can lead to more soreness in the muscles. For this reason, you should schedule it far enough from your peak workouts and races that it will not negatively affect your performance. Five days or more should do. Be sure to communicate openly with your massage therapist about your experience during deep tissue massage. Athletes are used to enduring discomfort; it is not in your best interest here. If you are fighting not to gasp, speak up! Otherwise you might find the massage that is intended to relax you leaves you more tense, sore, and even bruised.

You may find therapists who specialize in deep tissue or in Swedish massage; most will be trained and comfortable in both, so you need not feel that you have to commit to one or the other. A good massage therapist will draw on his or her experience to deliver what your body most needs. And as a good massage recipient, you'll let them know about your experience—what's working, what is not. Don't hold back.

Other Bodywork Modalities

Other bodywork modalities can complement your massage therapy work and your training. These techniques can have profound impact on your body, and thus should be slotted in the off-season or when an injury needs to be addressed.

Assisted Stretching

In assisted stretching, a practitioner aids the athlete in stretching through the full range of motion. An experienced practitioner will recognize imbalances and faulty movement patterns in the body and will work with the athlete in hands-on stretching, engaging and releasing the muscles, to bring the body into better balance. The Mattes method and the Whartons' approach, both versions of Active Isolated Stretching, are two examples. Thai yoga massage is another. This can be great for increasing your mobility and flexibility, potentially warding off imbalances that can lead to injury. Stretching does not seem to directly speed muscle recovery,[9] but that doesn't mean it's not useful and relaxing!

Myofascial Release

In myofascial release, the practitioner targets the fascia through gentle, targeted touch over long holds, with the goal of helping restructure the body from the fascia outward. This system can be helpful in addressing overuse injuries but is more therapeutic than recovery based, used to treat an injury or imbalance instead of simply working to help the body recover as a whole.

Structural Integration (Rolfing)

Structural Integration, like myofascial release, aims to restructure the body toward better alignment, but it uses a deeper touch. Massage therapist Leah Kangas explains, "This work is deep, often with big changes in the body. If someone is able to prioritize it, I would have this work done in the off-season or during a long recovery phase. This way as the body changes, time can be allowed for these changes to become familiar to the body without having to continue in an intense training cycle. However, if this work seems particularly helpful for someone, I won't hold off because they are in an intense cycle of training."

Depending on the practitioner, you may be advised to follow the round of 10 treatments designed by Ida Rolf, who popularized this modality, or you may be able to work directly on your individual needs. Either way, deep work like Structural Integration is best scheduled in the off-season, far from peak events.

Eastern Modalities

Other modalities, such as acupressure, acupuncture, dry needling, cupping, and Reiki (a Japanese form of energy work) may or may not be effective for recovery; these Eastern modalities are not well studied in the Western scientific literature. If you have the means and access to a practitioner, consider trying them out. Simply going through the motions of making time to focus on your well-being can, in and of itself, enhance your recovery.

WHEN TO SCHEDULE MASSAGE

I had the good fortune of coaching an athlete, Suzanna Dupee, who's a massage therapist. In researching the first edition of this book, I received massages weekly, sometimes more than one a week. While it's fantastic, especially during periods of work stress, it feels overly indulgent—even for me as a spa owner who conducts legitimate research on the market! I suspect a standard one or two massages a month would probably serve the same purpose for me.

Many athletes wonder about the timing of massage. How frequently should one get a massage, and if regular massage is not an option, when would be a good time to schedule one as an occasional treat? Timing depends on the point you have reached in the season and the proximity of key workouts and races.

Throughout the Season

How frequently you enjoy a massage will probably be dictated by your budget. While once a week would be nice, once a month is probably fine. This massage can go somewhere during your rest week or during a period of slightly reduced load. Since you might feel sore or slower the next day, be sure to schedule it away from long or hard workouts.

During my pregnancies, I enjoyed regular massages, scheduled to align with the frequency of my visits to my obstetrician-gynecologist. In the early stages, monthly visits and massages were appropriate; as I came closer to term, I went every third week, then biweekly, and then once a week until delivery. While I was preparing for an endurance event of a different kind, the frequency of my massages might give you an idea of how you can increase your visits but decrease their intensity as you approach your peak event. This works best if you are a massage regular and aware of how massage affects your body. And just as a pregnant woman would seek a therapist familiar with her special needs, you should look for a therapist familiar with athletes' needs.

If you are not getting regular massages, be careful scheduling a treatment too close to your peak event. Kangas explains, "I see people coming in the week before their race never having received a massage before. It might be helpful, but usually there is so much to work through so many layers, and of course you wouldn't want to make too much change at this point." Better to schedule the occasional massage farther from a race, ideally during a quiet period in your training. It will also avoid aggravating tissue that is already stressed.

Before and after a Race

As you approach your goal race or event, the type of massage should vary according to your competition schedule. In other words, when you're still farther from the race, you can receive deeper work; as you get closer to the event, a lighter touch is key.

Massage therapist Carolyn Levy divides the time line around a peak event into a few stages. First, three weeks from competition, she suggests a thorough, therapeutic massage to, in her words, "work all the kinks out." This massage, "deep and slow," as Levy describes it, can go in the two or three days after your peak workout of the preceding cycle. Levy will prescribe an ice bath later that evening, before bed. She warns her athletes that they will feel a little sluggish the next day but promises, "the body will swing back within 48 to 72 hours."

Three days before the event, Levy will massage the athlete using a lighter touch at a faster pace. The goal in this lighter massage is to pass through the muscle tissues, helping them flush and refresh. If you take a day of rest in your race week, the massage could go on that day or precede it. Just keep it a day or two removed from your event itself—farther if it's a very big event. Tim DeBoom says, "Before an Ironman, I'll get my last body work done about four days before the race. I always feel pretty crappy the day after body work, so I try to have plenty of time to absorb it before a big race."

Immediately after the event itself, Levy suggests a brief massage, "a good 10-minute flush-out, and some stretching," which she feels signals to the body to begin its repair work. If you visit the massage tent after a race, be sure that your experience is a relaxing one. This is not the time to add aggravation to already inflamed tissue.

A few days after the event, another light massage is in order to book-end the one scheduled a few days before the event. Levy says the intention is "flushing, not terribly deep. You don't want to traumatize the tissue, but again to deliver the message that you can open up."

Finally, within a week or so, the body will be ready for a return to its normal massage schedule.

In a Day

Whenever possible, schedule your massage for later in the day, after your workout. It can be especially restful—if not financially practical—to have your therapist travel to your home, so that you don't have to drive after your treatment and can instead continue relaxing.

If you must schedule a massage before a workout, try to make it an easy workout, and assume that you will feel different from usual. It's probably not the best time to go out and run technical trail.

WHEN NOT TO SCHEDULE MASSAGE

A quick word of caution: Massage may be palliative care for an injury, as it helps you feel better all over. But booking a massage is not the same as scheduling an appointment with a sports-medicine specialist or physical therapist. If you have pain related to training, be sure you are addressing the cause of the trouble by having your symptoms and biomechanics evaluated. Be honest with yourself; take a good, hard look at your training and recovery. Don't use massage as a Band-Aid.

HOW TO FIND A MASSAGE THERAPIST

Massage licensure laws vary among countries, and within countries, they vary among states and provinces. In the United States, not all states regulate massage therapists. Most states require state licensure; a few require state certification; a few are unregulated. A quick search online will explain the law in your area and unearth a few directories to help you find a local practitioner. Don't be shy about asking for a potential therapist's credentials. Look at the amount of hours the therapist has trained. Six hundred hours or more of training are a good sign; a weekend certification is not. Better still is a therapist with additional training in working with athletes.

Beyond licensure and certification, you are looking for a massage therapist who understands your body and needs as an athlete. Ideally, he or she is not only experienced in working with athletes of your sport but also actively engaging in that sport. Such a person will be sympathetic and will understand not only the athlete's body but also the athlete's psyche. Kangas cautions, "Many therapists don't understand athletes and their drive, and will often develop a mindset: 'Well, if you just didn't do so much (insert activity here).' Also, a therapist with experience working with athletes of your particular activity will have that much more experience in working with similar injuries and imbalances."

The best way to locate a therapist in your area is through referrals. Ask your training partners, local running and bike store workers, and local sports-medicine practitioners for their recommendations. But remember, tastes are very individual, so you'll want to try the therapist for yourself and to communicate clearly about your needs, including the type of pressure you prefer. One person's torture hour is another person's deep release.

Prices for massage vary, depending on area and venue. Expect to pay more at a luxury spa and less at a franchise such as Massage Envy or Hand and Stone. These outfits operate on a membership/subscription model that can bring the price down to a point where massage can be a regular part of your self-care routine. And remember, price doesn't always correlate to quality. If you find a provider who helps you feel better, and it's in your budget, rebook!

THE BOTTOM LINE

Massage can be a productive, relaxing, and enjoyable part of your training regimen. Depending on your budget and needs, it might be an occasional treat or an important routine. As with the other modalities described here, find what works for you and your budget. Personally, I suggest a monthly massage, with more frequent massages during peak volume weeks and closer to the race. Committing to self-care and relaxation through massage is a good first step toward building in more time for recovery and restoration.

QUICK TIPS

- Communication is key: Ask your massage therapist about his or her experience working with athletes, and tell your massage therapist about your needs, likes, and dislikes.
- Space more vigorous body work farther away from your peak events.
- The benefits of massage extend beyond the physical because receiving a massage gives you a chance to take a mental break.

Self-Massage

> **Time:** low to moderate
>
> **Cost:** low to moderate
>
> **Accessibility:** great
>
> **Confidence:** high
>
> **Contraindications:** overdoing self-massage and irritating inflamed tissue

Massage is a popular and important tool for recovery, but it can quickly get prohibitively expensive. If you don't have the luxury of regular massage, you can bridge the gap between sessions with some self-massage. Self-massage helps you release adhesions, knots, and trigger points in the soft tissues and is an important part of injury prevention. It is also a way to give yourself some assistance in stretches, by anchoring one end of a muscle against the ground, your hand, or a device while you stretch in the other direction. Since the body works as a kinetic chain, self-massage can target every link.

Scientific evidence supporting the use of self-massage is mixed, but an umbrella review of the existing literature concludes that there are no negative effects of self–myofascial release, or SMR—another way to describe self-massage—beyond any pain experienced during the actual massage.[1] Happily, this sensation is completely within each athlete's control. One 2014 study showed that self-massage with a foam roller reduced athletes' muscle soreness in the days after using the roller, which is promising.[2] A recent review of all the literature on rolling suggests that it may be more beneficial as a way to improve mobility before a workout than as a means to enhance recovery after a workout.[3] Still, any activity that gets you tuned in to your body, breathing deeply, and resting low to the ground is probably a good way to start a positive spiral of recovery habits.

Ultrarunner Keith Straw recommends manipulating any area in the body that is bothering you. "I do a lot of poking around myself," he says. "I prod my knees, rub my feet, pound my pecs." USA Cycling *soigneur* Bernard Condevaux advises self-massage as well. "There's an economic reality, and a lot of teams can't afford *soigneurs* or individual massage," he says. To get the most from your self-massage on a foam roller, he suggests, "Be aware of what you're doing. Keep it moving. Roll toward your heart. If you find a spot that's tight or tender, sit on it for 10 seconds. If it doesn't back off, change the pressure. Mashing the muscle is not always the best thing. The target is flushing out, getting the muscle to recover, not beating it."

TOOLS

Your hands are the simplest tool for self-massage. Reach into areas of the body that are calling for your attention and see if you can feel what's going on. Trace the muscle fibers to their origin and insertion points, along either end. Is there a particular sore spot or trigger point? How does it respond to pressure?

Applying cross-friction massage, against the grain of the muscle fibers, can help release adhesions and scar tissue limiting your range of motion.

Other devices include foam rollers, beaded sticks, balls, and branded devices, such as Trigger Point Therapy devices. Let's examine what to look for in your tools.

Foam rollers come in various densities and durabilities. The simplest is a white Styrofoam roller, similar to a floating noodle pool toy (but thicker) and widely available. The foam has some give, keeping the massage a little lighter than a denser roller. They are inexpensive but may not last long. Also available are darker rollers made of high-density foam. Even more rigid are rollers with foam or a material with protuberant nubs wrapped around a hard core.

Vibrating rollers are covered in foam, and typically have a vibrating feature that can be dialed up or down. A 2019 study showed that versus nonvibrating rollers, vibrating rollers decreased pain perception in athletes, while also increasing range of motion in the hip joint. While the latter isn't related to recovery, perception of postexercise pain may be. Note that the study measured immediate perception of pain, not how athletes felt a day or two after. And, of course, you can't blind athletes as to whether the roller is vibrating or nonvibrating. But if you enjoy a vibrating roller over a nonvibrating one, there's no reason not to use it.[4]

Beaded sticks feature hard plastic or wooden beads on a stick. The shape and material of the beads will affect your experience; if possible, try the implement out before buying.

Balls from various sports make useful, inexpensive self-massage devices. Golf balls work well for the bottoms of the feet, as do small hard rubber balls (think Superball). Lacrosse balls or baseballs (even softballs or their rubber substitutes) work into the calves and deep hip rotators. Tennis balls can be good choices, depending on their firmness and the sensitivity of the area being worked. Two balls lashed together with athletic tape make a peanut shape that's especially useful for working the muscles on either side of the spine.

You can get creative as you choose your implements. Elite runner Marc Jeuland uses a wooden rolling pin for self-massage. Ultramarathoner Nikki Kimball uses an antler!

TECHNIQUE AND TIME

The general technique for using any of these implements is similar. Put the device on the floor, place your leg or arm or back on it, and apply pressure (or place a ball between your body and the wall, if you're working your chest and back muscles and want less intensity). Once the pressure feels right, slowly travel along the muscle fibers a few times, pausing as you feel particular points of tightness. In general, you will move distally to centrally—in other words, making trips from the periphery of the body toward the center. If it feels productive to travel back and forth along the muscle from end to end, that is fine, too.

You can work the whole body or just problem areas such as the plantar fasciae on the bottom of the feet and the iliotibial (IT) band. A few passes over each muscle or area should do. More is not always better! If your muscles are already inflamed or overtired, overdoing your self-massage will simply aggravate the condition and prevent your recovery—yielding a result opposite from what you intended. Bigger muscle groups can probably take more pressure than smaller groups. Let your body be your guide.

How often you do self-massage depends on your time, schedule, and needs. It might become a nightly habit, part of your downtime ritual. Or maybe you take care to do your self-massage on the days when you run long or hard—or just on the days when you run, if you are a multisport athlete. Experiment to find what works best for you.

SELF-MASSAGE FOR COMMON PROBLEMS

Quadriceps

The four large muscles of the quadriceps are a good starting point for your foam rolling. Take a leg to one edge of your roller, with the other leg resting on the ground. You'll be resting on your palms or elbows. Start with the roller positioned just above your knee and slowly push your hips back so that you roll in toward the center along the front of your thigh. After a few passes here, turn to the outer edge of your leg. (You can bend your supporting leg at the knee and have the sole of the foot on the ground.) Follow with some long strokes up the inner quadriceps muscles (figure 15.1).

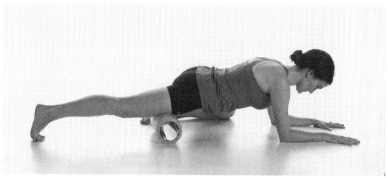

FIGURE 15.1
Quadriceps. © *Steve Clarke*

Hamstrings

Sit your bottom on the ground, with the back of one or both legs resting on the roller just above the back of the knee. Supporting weight in your hands, slowly roll your hips toward the roller. After a few trips, rotate to the outer and inner edges of the hamstrings (figure 15.2).

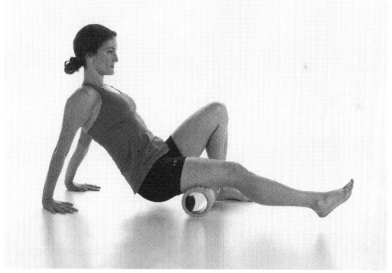

FIGURE 15.2
Hamstrings. © *Steve Clarke*

Calves

You'll work on your calves in much the same way as the hamstrings, rolling up and down slowly and taking care to get to both edges as well as the central musculature. You may find, however, that the weight of your lower leg and foot isn't heavy enough to give the same massage. Add weight by crossing one ankle over the other and focusing your attention on the bottom leg (figure 15.3).

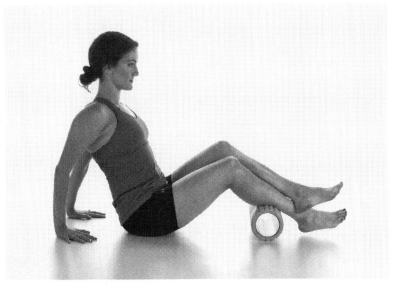

FIGURE 15.3
Calves. © *Steve Clarke*

Iliotibial (IT) Band

Working your IT band can be an excruciating experience. Check that you are not going too deep; if you are gasping, you may be forcing the issue, which can aggravate existing inflammation.

Sit one hip on the roller, with the other leg bent at the knee, sole of the foot on the floor. If you're rolling your right leg, your right hand or elbow will rest on the floor. Start at the bottom of the thigh, just outside and above the knee, and slowly make your way toward the outer hip (figure 15.4). You may have to pause to breathe deeply and collect yourself— again, be sure you aren't working too hard. A few passes should suffice.

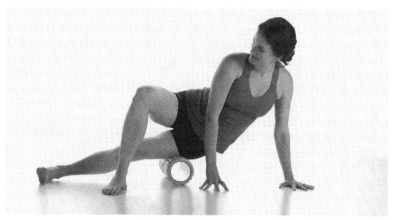

FIGURE 15.4
Iliotibial band. © *Steve Clarke*

Outer Hip

Continuing upward from your IT band work, explore the muscles of the outer hip (figure 15.5). Your gluteal muscles are prime targets, as is the piriformis muscle, which lies deep in the hip. If you can't reach deep enough with the roller, use a tennis ball or a harder, rubber ball. You'll sit on it, lean back into your hands, and explore until you find the right spot.

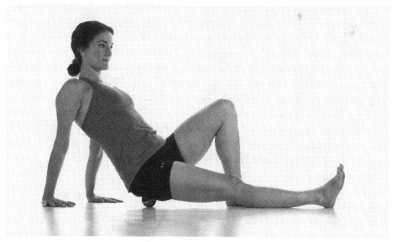

FIGURE 15.5
Outer hip. © *Steve Clarke*

Soles of the Feet

The plantar fasciae that run along the bottoms of your feet are prime territory to explore with a smaller implement, be it a tennis ball, rubber ball, or a golf ball. If you're using a softer device, you may be able to stand and carefully place your body weight onto the ball. If it's a harder device such as a golf ball, you'll want to sit down so that the sensation doesn't grow too intense. Roll over both the arch, from the heel to the ball of the foot, and the spaces between the metatarsals, running the ball into the four spaces at the base of the five toes (figure 15.6).

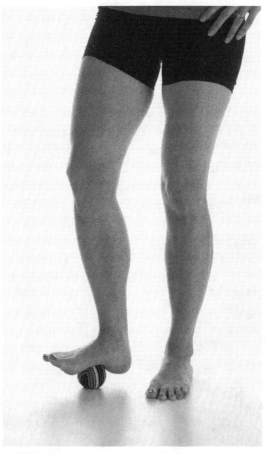

FIGURE 15.6
Soles of the feet. © Steve Clarke

Back

Use the roller to run up and down your back, finding spots that need extra attention (figure 15.7). If certain areas are particularly sore, you may want to revisit them with a smaller implement, such as a tennis or rubber ball. Two balls taped together can work right along either edge of the spine. Go slowly and pay attention to your experience. Breathe deeply into the places where sensation is the strongest.

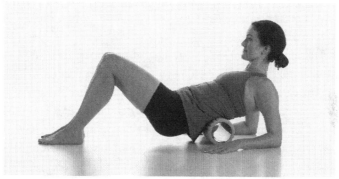

FIGURE 15.7
Back. © *Steve Clarke*

Chest

Depending on the size and shape of your chest (and the size and shape of your breasts), you may have success lying face-down on the roller (figure 15.8). If that's infeasible, use a smaller, handheld ball. Hold the ball against the pectoralis muscles as you roll, or if you need greater force, take the ball to the corner of a wall and work in from there.

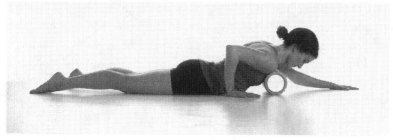

FIGURE 15.8
Chest. © *Steve Clarke*

PASSIVE SELF-MASSAGE DEVICES

Air Compression Devices

NormaTec is a compression device originally created by Dr. Laura Jacobs for rehabilitation of patients with vascular disease and later adapted for use in sports recovery. The device consists of sleeves for the limbs (arms or legs) and a computer-controlled compressor. The athlete rests while the system applies the patented peristaltic pulse (wavelike) dynamic compression to the limb to maximize circulation. You can now find similar products offered by Therabody and a range of other outfits at various price levels.

Physiologist Bill Sands says that apart from smart training, rest, and a good diet, the NormaTec MVP Pro is the best recovery tool available. He explains that static compression, like that applied by compression garments, is much less powerful for enhancing recovery than dynamic compression. Dynamic compression helps pump lymph out of the swollen, edematous tissues where it accumulates. In addition, he says, peristaltic compression will reduce inflammation. While massage can help, Sands says, "it's hard to encircle an entire limb with your hands. It'll make you feel better, but it won't enhance performance."

If you have the means to use one of these machines, do. Many athletes from pros to age groupers have raved to me about their benefits.

Massage Guns

Massage guns offer a percussive massage that sends the head of the device, which can be covered in attachments of various shapes and sizes, against the body. Depending on an athlete's sensitivity and massage preferences, this can be pleasant or excruciating. There is a danger of overdoing it with a massage gun. In one extreme case, an athlete suffered rhabdomyolysis—extreme muscle damage—after use of the massage gun.[5] Matt Driller of La Trobe University and the Australian Institute of Sport has begun research into the guns but says, "At the moment, I don't encourage the use of massage guns as a recovery strategy, as I need to see a bit more evidence of their efficacy first." If you are a fan, use it with some caution, and remember that less may be more. Driller says that their initial findings, along with similar findings from other groups, "found increases in muscle soreness after using a massage gun." Thus despite massage guns' popularity in recent years, there is a lot more that needs to be studied. They may be best used sparingly and when you don't have a big workout scheduled shortly after use. Better guidelines may also be needed on their application: firmness, setting, use of attachments.

QUICK TIPS

- Self-massage can bridge the gaps between regular sessions with a massage therapist or might replace paying a massage therapist entirely.

- Smaller balls such as golf or tennis balls can work into smaller muscles; foam rollers (or even rolling pins) can work larger muscles.

- Don't be too aggressive: A few passes over each of the major muscle groups should suffice.

- If you find yourself routinely revisiting a problem spot, check that your body is balanced biomechanically and that you have the right work/rest balance in your training.

16

Restorative Yoga

> **Time:** low to moderate
>
> **Cost:** free to low (for props)
>
> **Accessibility:** great
>
> **Confidence:** high
>
> **Contraindications:** injury to the back; modify poses as needed

As a yoga teacher and practitioner as well as a coach, I have spent years seeing how yoga enhances my recovery and the recovery of athletes I teach and coach. Several of my other books detail the ways yoga enhances training. But yoga can also be used very specifically as a restorative practice to directly improve recovery. It must be done carefully, though. The 21st-century West offers a multitude of approaches to yoga, from the very gentle to the very intense and hot and everything in between. Attending a class that is too intense may interfere with your recovery at best and could lead to injury at worst, especially if you are the competitive type. Look for a restorative class or follow the guidelines here for home practice.

158

WHICH KINDS OF YOGA HASTEN RECOVERY

To encourage your recovery, choose styles that are breath focused, relaxing, and slow. They'll have titles including keywords like *gentle* or *quiet*. Restorative yoga is a fantastic choice. In restorative poses, the focus is not on strengthening or even on stretching but instead on releasing tension. This is part of what makes it perfect as a recovery practice. While other forms of yoga can be great for improving mobility, flexibility, strength, and self-awareness, stretching doesn't seem to have a direct, measurable effect on muscular recovery. A 2021 meta-analysis of randomized controlled trials on the benefits of stretching for recovery shows no evidence that stretching hastens recovery.[1] Restorative yoga is not about stretching. Restorative poses are held for a long while—10 or 15 minutes or even more—and are fully supported by props, including bolsters, blankets, sandbags, and the floor. As you release into the props, you'll relax your body, your breath, and your mind.

The gentle inversions of restorative yoga, especially the legs-up-the-wall pose (*viparita karani*, in Sanskrit), will help drain edema from the legs. Sometimes this is a very noticeable experience, such as after a long or hard workout, when you can feel the shift of fluids back in toward the center. Sometimes it's more subtle. Among the other subtle effects are a shift in hormone levels in the body and the dilation of blood vessels in the upper body. These restorative poses will help your entire back settle down, releasing the tension that accumulates during the course of your workout and your day, and they will help broaden your chest, undoing the closing off that happens when your hands are on the handlebars, the keyboard, or the steering wheel, and recreating space for your breath.

In a restorative pose, you'll have plenty of time to be still and notice your breath. Let it flow freely in and out, expanding your belly, your ribcage, and your upper chest on inhalation and leaving your upper chest, your ribcage, and your belly on exhalation. Let your breath be the focus of your awareness. This focus—on relaxation—can be tough, though. Ultrarunner Charlie Engle admits, "When I go into that yoga class, even the relaxing is hard for me; that's my personality. It takes full concentration to do yoga, while running is mindless for me. It's actually harder than running." If your thoughts drift to other subjects, notice, and turn your attention back to your breath. This will elicit the relaxation response (see chapter 17 for more) as well as improve your ability to focus.

You don't need to be "doing yoga" for the benefits of a restorative practice to work. Many athletes arrive at a restorative process spontaneously, by listening to their bodies. Ultrarunner Keith Straw, who holds a 24-hour personal record of 137 miles, has a mantra: "When I run, I run. When I'm not running, I rest." He says, "I spend hours lying down with my legs draped over a yoga ball watching reruns of *Law and Order*." This simple approach to inversion can work wonders.

Former *Runner's World* editor and ultrarunner Jennifer Van Allen testifies to the benefits of yoga: "I feel it's an integral part of my ability to recover." She believes yoga keeps her muscles loose and supple and increases their pliability. "I feel yoga is a preventative way to jumpstart the recovery process," she says.

WHAT YOU NEED

Here are some restorative poses you can do at home. For the full experience, you'll want to gather props to support yourself. These props include a few blankets or beach towels, a pillow or two, and an eye bag (a lightly weighted pillow to cover your eyes, widely available). Blocks can be handy risers to boost the height of your bolsters. A yoga strap can be useful, too. If you have access to a sandbag (you can buy them online), it can add to your experience of settling in. Handy people can sew their own sandbag by making an envelope about 6 inches by 18 inches and inserting a sealed plastic bag filled with playground sand from the hardware store.

You'll need quiet space for your yoga practice. Ideally, you'll be away from electronics, which can beep and distract you, and out of view of your home office, pets, and children.

Finally, you'll need a timer. A kitchen timer works, but it can have a harsh alarm sound. Various alarms on cell phones might work better. If you can set a chime to ring every five minutes, you'll be able to count off your time and to change the position of your head in poses where you're face down. The timer will keep you in the pose for the right amount of time, and it will wake you up should you fall asleep. It may also help you relax, knowing the timer is running and that you don't need to pay attention to how long you've been in a pose. Instead, you'll focus on just being in the pose, breathing, and letting go.

POSES

The poses described here can be strung together in order to make a full routine. (You'll find it demonstrated at sagerountree.com/recovery.) Or choose the ones that feel best for you to create a shorter practice. When you practice the full routine, you'll take your spine through six planes of motion: forward folding, backward bending, side bending in either direction, and twisting in either direction. When creating a shorter practice, be sure to balance any forward folding with backward bending and to twist or side bend to both sides until you feel even.

In each of these, you're looking for the sensation of comfort and support—not a deep stretch. Just as your active recovery workouts should be very light, so should your restorative yoga poses. If you make it too intense, you are changing from a restorative practice to a flexibility practice, just as working too hard in an active recovery workout changes it to an endurance workout.

Legs Up the Wall

For legs up the wall, you'll need a wall or a closed and locked door. Having a stack of a few blankets, a roll of towels, or a yoga bolster can enhance the pose.

At its simplest, the pose will take an L shape, with your back against the floor and your legs up the wall (figure 16.1). Getting there can be tricky. Sit with one hip against the wall, then swing yourself around so

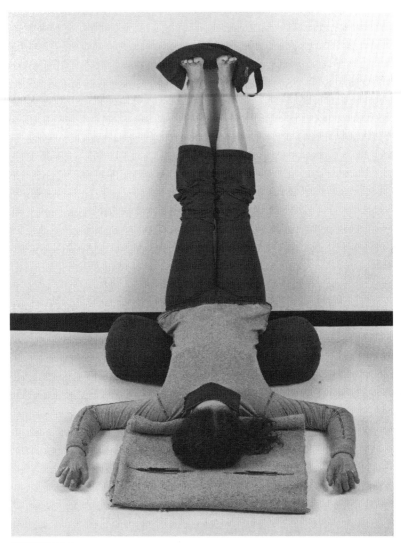

FIGURE 16.1
Legs up the wall. © *Steve Clarke*

that your spine rests on the floor and your legs are propped on the wall. If your hamstrings allow, scoot your bottom all the way to the wall or baseboard. If you find your hamstrings are tight, you can keep your bottom a few inches from the wall, but to be sure you aren't hyperextending your knees, keep them in a slight bend. Take your arms to a position that feels comfortable. This could be an inverted V, out to a T, in an open Y overhead, or split into a W. Wherever your arms are, roll your palms toward the ceiling to help open your chest and shoulders.

If you have props on hand, you can make this pose into a gentle supported backbend. Lay your bolster, pillow, or a rectangular folded blanket so its longer end runs parallel to the wall and a few inches away from it. Sitting on the prop, slide your legs up the wall and let your entire pelvis rest on the cushion. The prop should support your lower back fully while stretching your ribcage. If you feel like you've got too strong a curve in your neck, add a rolled blanket under your head. If you have an eye bag, try putting it over your eyes or simply on your forehead. If you have a sandbag, it can rest on top of your feet to settle your legs toward the ground. (You can start with it as you push your legs up the wall, or have a friend add it once you're in place.)

Stay in this position for a good while—10 minutes or up to 20, if you can. Should your legs fall asleep, simply bend your knees toward your chest for a few breaths and reposition them. If your legs won't stay together, you can use a yoga strap to tie them together loosely. This is a good place to experiment with economy of form. Use only as much energy as you need to hold your legs up the wall. Try relaxing entirely. Worst-case scenario: Your legs will slide down the wall, and you'll have to reposition them. Not a problem!

Legs on a Chair

A variation on legs up the wall involves placing your calves on the seat of a chair, on a sofa, or on a coffee table (figure 16.2). Bending the knees will alleviate strain on the back, so this is a nice option if your lower back or knees don't do well in a full version of legs up the wall.

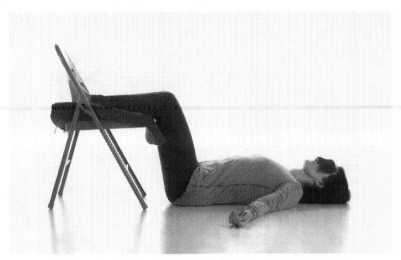

FIGURE 16.2
Legs on a chair. © *Steve Clarke*

Depending on the length of your femurs, you may need to add some padding to the support beneath your calves. Make sure your back is resting happily on the ground and improvise with props if you feel they will support your relaxation here. A stay of 10 minutes or more is ideal, and an eye bag is a nice touch.

Supported Child's Pose

In supported child's pose, you'll get a release for your low back and a gentle stretch for your hamstrings, quadriceps, and shins (figure 16.3). Remember, this should be only the gentlest of stretches; prop yourself up if it feels too intense, especially if the intensity is in your knees.

With a bolster running vertically in front of you and some padding beneath your legs (this could be carpeting, a yoga mat, or a blanket), take your knees wide while keeping your big toes together. Holding your hips over your heels, lean your belly to the support and settle in. If you feel too much of a stretch, add a layer or two to the support. You can also add a blanket between your calves and thighs, to alleviate

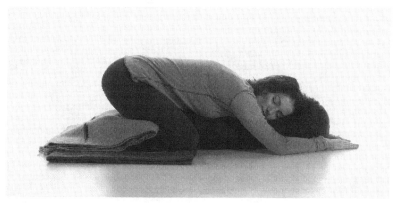

FIGURE 16.3
Supported child's pose. © *Steve Clarke*

pressure on the knees. If a friend is on hand to help you, have him or her place the sandbag across the back of your pelvis.

Start with one side of your head on the bolster, and after five minutes, turn to the other side. Your timer can help you here, especially if you can set an interim chime. When the timer goes off, turn your head to the second side, and when it goes off again, either stay for another interval or move to another pose.

Supported Prone Twist

The supported prone twist is a lovely pose that wrings tension from the spine while offering a gentle stretch to the outer hip, enhanced by the weight of the body sinking into the pose (figure 16.4). To take this shape, sit on one hip, knees bent and touching, with a bolster or stack of blankets running perpendicular to your thighs. Take your hands to either side of the bolster, draw your spine long, and then slowly lower your belly down to the support. You might prop yourself up on your elbows, depending on the height of your props, or you could place your arms anywhere that feels comfortable.

As with supported child's pose, you can choose how to position your head. Facing in the same direction as your legs will give you a more

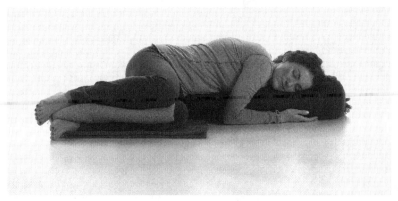

FIGURE 16.4
Supported prone twist. © *Steve Clarke*

gentle experience. Turning your head away from your legs will give a fuller twist but might feel too intense. Let your body and your breath be your guide. If your chosen position causes any stress or strain or affects your breathing, you'll need to change and reposition yourself into a more comfortable position. Spending at least 5 minutes here is good; 10 minutes is better. Repeat the pose on the other side when you are done with the first.

Supported Supine Twist

The supported supine twist will take you sunny-side-up. While it will affect your hips less than the supported prone twist, it will encourage more openness in your chest. Lie on your back with a bolster or folded blanket on either side of you. Reach one leg long and bend the other, dropping the inner knee of this bent leg to the pillow at your side. You'll roll all the way to the hip of the straight leg (figure 16.5).

Check that this position is gentle and relaxing. If it is, reach your arms into a T position, propping one or both of them on blankets if that feels best. As with the previous twist, you can turn your head either way, or simply face up with a neutral neck position for 5–10 minutes.

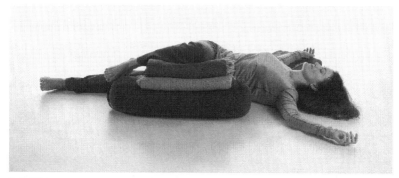

FIGURE 16.5
Supported supine twist. © *Steve Clarke*

Supported Backbend

If you have time for only one restorative yoga pose in a day, the supported backbend (figure 16.6) makes a good choice. (And if you have time for two, couple this with legs up the wall.)

It's worth taking the time to carefully set up your supported backbend, so that you can receive maximum benefits from this wonderfully

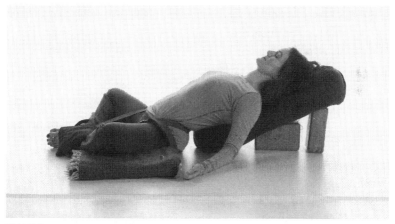

FIGURE 16.6
Supported backbend. © *Steve Clarke*

restorative position. It will undo the hunch so many of us carry from our desk jobs and our training, it will create space across the chest and ribcage for freer breathing, and its open-hearted position will be deeply relaxing and affirming.

If you have a block or two on hand, set them into a T position so that they can prop up one end of your bolster. Sit your hips at the other end, and recline against the bolster. Your head will be slightly elevated, but your chin can stay low. Spread your arms out. If they dangle in space, support them on pillows or blankets.

Your legs could rest in a number of different positions here. If your lower back feels tender, keep your knees bent and the soles of your feet on the floor. You could even support them from below, if you have enough props. If your back isn't complaining, you can stretch your legs long in front of you. Or, for a gentle release of the inner thighs, take the soles of the feet together, knees bent, and drop your knees to either side, ideally onto cushions. If you like this leg position (*baddha konasana*, bound angle pose, often called "cobbler") but your legs are sliding away from you, you can hold them steady by draping a sand bag across your feet. Alternatively, loosely tie them together by taking your strap behind your back, over your thighs and calves, and under your feet. The strap can connect over one thigh, so you can adjust it tighter or looser with a hand. Stay in this supported backbend for as long as you can, up to 20 minutes.

Supported Side Bend

Taking a very gentle lateral stretch over your bolster will release the musculature around your shoulders and open the intercostal muscles between your ribs, creating more space for breathing (figure 16.7).

Rest on one hip with a pile of blankets, or a bolster and a blanket, at your side. Lay the side of your body onto this support as you stretch both arms overhead, like a synchronized swimmer taking a side dive into the water. Your palms can meet, or you can hold the wrist of the top arm with the hand of the bottom arm. Your head relaxes against

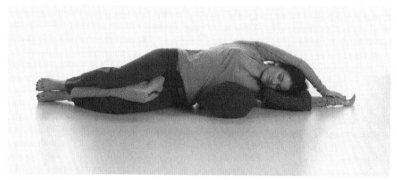

FIGURE 16.7
Supported side bend. © *Steve Clarke*

the inside of your upper arm or against a support, if you prefer. Stay
here for five or more minutes, practicing relaxed but deep breathing,
expanding your ribcage. Then repeat on the second side.

Supported Bridge

Bridge pose is an important pose for athletes, and it is often prescribed in physical therapy. It stretches the hip flexors, engages the
hamstrings and gluteal muscles, and strengthens the back muscles. This
version (figure 16.8), a supported one, requires no muscular energy. It
will open the chest in a gentle backbend, giving the hip flexors time to
release slowly.

You can do this pose using a yoga block or a pillow. Each will yield
a slightly different experience. To use the block, lie on your back with
your knees bent and your feet close to your sit-bones. Lift your hips and
place the block horizontally underneath your pelvis—an inch or two
below the waistband is probably the right place. Start with the block at
medium height and lift it higher only if you feel really supported there.
You can walk your feet away from you if that feels good. Stay for a few
minutes, letting your chest open and your hip flexors release. When you
are ready to move on, lift your hips, remove the block, and spend a few
breaths resting flat on the floor.

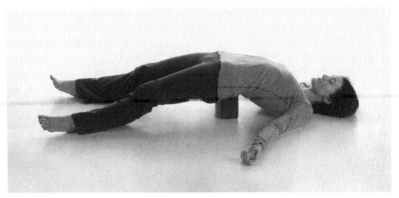

FIGURE 16.8
Supported bridge. © *Steve Clarke*

To rest on the pillow, lay it vertically along your spine and slide back until your shoulder blades are on the ground and your ribcage is spreading. The pillow should support you from the midback to the pelvis. If your legs won't stay in a neutral position, you can lay a sandbag over them or strap them together. Rest your arms alongside the pillow, palms up. Stay for a few minutes, and when you are done, slide backward off the pillow and rest on the floor for a few breaths.

Supported Corpse Pose

Corpse pose offers a wonderful position for rest: It is the ultimate do-nothing position. While it is traditionally practiced lying flat on the ground, adding props can make it a more restful experience and will keep you comfortable for longer (figure 16.9).

Adding a support beneath your knees or calves (a bolster or a folded or rolled blanket) will help your lower back settle into the ground. Experiment with these two different positions: With the support under your knees, your heels can touch the ground; with the support under your calves, your heels may hang in the air.

A sandbag placed horizontally across the pelvis, a few inches beneath the waist, can provide comforting weight. Lighter weights can help keep

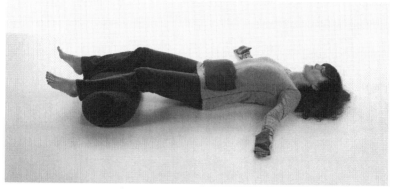

FIGURE 16.9
Supported corpse pose. © *Steve Clarke*

the fingers spread as the palms face upward; an eye bag can do the trick. An
eye bag, on your eyes or spread across your forehead, is also a nice touch.
Finally, consider a light pillow or a few thicknesses of folded blanket.

Once everything is set up, stay here for a good long while. In yoga,
we use this rule of thumb: Take 5–10 minutes of corpse pose for every
hour of physical practice. This works for training, too. If you've finished
a three-hour session, 30 minutes of restorative yoga, including corpse
pose, will help you feel relaxed and balanced.

QUICK TIPS

- Restorative poses, held for 5–20 minutes at a time, give
  your body and mind a chance to relax and begin restoration.
- A quiet room and a few props will enhance your restorative yoga experience.
- The more restless you feel, the more you need to stay
  and relax.

17

Meditation and Breathing

> **Time:** low to moderate
>
> **Cost:** free
>
> **Accessibility:** great
>
> **Confidence:** high
>
> **Contraindications:** none

Meditation, whether done in conjunction with a practice of yoga poses or as a stand-alone event, gives you the time and space to see things as they are. An increased awareness of the state of your being will help you become aware of the state of your recovery and will show you when you need to take another easy day, as well as when you are ready to push. Such self-awareness will help you avoid overtraining and reach peak performance. Many of the elite athletes I've talked with say they don't really track their metrics per se; they "just know" when they are tired and need a little time off. Matt Fitzgerald's book *Run: The Mind-Body Method of Running by Feel* is full of similar anecdotes and explains how to rely on your intuition as you train.[1] Meditation can help develop your intuition by building your mindfulness about the state of your body and your life in the present moment. The more honed your self-awareness, the better you can understand the state of your body's recovery and can thus push when you are ready and pull back when you need rest. Although it need not be a conscious contemplation of your goals, meditation can give you the clarity and the tools to check your goals and confirm that they are appropriate for you and the stage you have reached in training, career, relationships, and life.

Research at the School of Medicine at the University of California–Los Angeles shows that long-term meditators exhibit changes in the structure of their brains.[2] These changes to the orbito-frontal and hippocampal regions increase meditators' control of positive emotions and emotional stability—important attributes for athletes. Other research at Stanford University, Massachusetts General Hospital, the University of North Carolina–Chapel Hill, and the University of Michigan demonstrates behavioral effects: Subjects who practice meditation feel better, more focused, and more mindful.[3]

Meditation and breathing exercises will enhance your recovery. Physically, even taking a few minutes to sit down and scan your body will help remove tension from the muscles and making space for improved blood flow. Meditation and breathing exercises calm your central nervous system, helping you feel more relaxed, undoing some of the negative physiological effects of stressful training and life. And psychologically, meditation and careful breathing will help you feel calm and in control. Meditation and breathing exercises can also enhance your endurance, by giving you tools to remain attentive even when your body is aching or your mind is agitated.

SIMPLE MEDITATION TECHNIQUES

There are myriad approaches to meditation, with both religious and nonreligious origins. You need no particular faith to meditate beyond a faith in the process itself. And this faith is important because meditation is hard. We're constantly learning about the distracted state of our own minds, brought face-to-face with how they jump from thought to thought. This is not a problem; it is the process itself. Our goal is an awareness of the nature of our minds, not a complete silencing of them. We perceive the tumultuous state of our minds, but we don't engage with these roiling thoughts. Instead, we return to the task at hand, whether it be concentration or observation.

Here are three simple approaches to meditation. They will all work to enhance your awareness of your body and mind, so each will work for recovery. You might start with the counting meditation, as it is very accessible. Once you are comfortable with that, move on to mantra meditation or simply sitting in awareness and observation. For each of these approaches, you'll want to find a comfortable seat. If sitting on a cushion on the floor works for you, fantastic. You can sit cross-legged or in the "easy sit" position from yoga, in which your knees go wide and your heels line up with the midline of your body (figure 17.1). Or kneel with a yoga block supporting your sitting bones like a cruiser bike

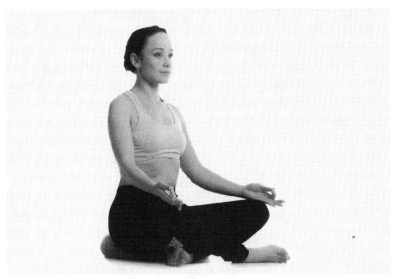

FIGURE 17.1
Sitting with your hips elevated should greatly increase your comfort in meditation. *Getty Images/fizkes*

saddle. If your hips are tight, your knees twinge, or your back aches, sit in a chair. Just be sure you are upright, instead of leaning back in the chair, so that you don't strain your back. You can keep your eyes open and focus a soft gaze on the wall or the floor, or you can close your eyes. It's generally a good idea not to lie down. If you're too comfortable, you'll fall asleep, and while sleep is crucial to your recovery, meditation is about consciousness, not unconsciousness. Of course, if you can't stay awake, sleep may be more important than meditation.

Aim to sit for a predetermined length of time, so that you don't give up at the first hint of difficulty. (It will be tough; expect a challenge.) Five minutes is a good starting point, and you can build to 20 or even 30. From there, you might add a second meditation each day. Working on weekly volume, you could try meditating each day for X minutes, where X is the number of hours you train per week. If you can't make time to meditate daily, aim for four or five days a week. I've found the benefits of a daily 20-minute sitting meditation to be very deep, bringing me greater presence of mind and equanimity during workouts, races, and life.

Counting Meditation

Counting meditation makes a good starting point as you begin a meditation practice. There are all kinds of patterns you can use. As you get started, try counting down from 30 to 1, assigning a number to each inhalation and each exhalation. Thus, you'd inhale and think, 30, and exhale thinking 29. With the next round of breath, count 28 and 27, and continue until you reach 1. You'll probably find yourself distracted before you get to single digits, and that's normal. Just go back to 30 and start again.

Once the countdown is easy, you can advance by starting from a higher number or by assigning a number to a complete round of inhalation and exhalation. Thus, you'd inhale 30 and exhale 30, inhale 29 and exhale 29, and so on. Eventually, you'll get to 1 and can sit, internally repeating 1 or dropping the counting entirely.

Alternatively, count up from 1 to 10 and repeat. Or count by fives, or count down from 100. The numbers aren't important: What matters is the task of focusing your mind, catching it when it wanders, and redirecting it to the work at hand.

Mantra Meditation

The Relaxation Response, Dr. Herbert Benson's breakthrough bestseller on the effect of meditation on the mind and body, prescribes a very simple and highly effective, clinically proven approach to meditation.[4] Benson's directions are to choose a "word, sound, phrase, prayer, or muscular activity" and to repeat it from a relaxed position without attachment to outcome. When you are distracted, passively notice that and return to the repetition.

This form of mantra meditation is loosely based on the technique of Transcendental Meditation, whose practitioners Benson studied. While the Transcendental Meditation approach involves the personal assignment of a secret mantra, or phrase, for repetition, Benson found that any word would do. Words that carry personal meaning can be especially useful, as they will hold your attention longer than abstract neutral words or phrases. Benson suggests simply repeating "One." You might choose a word like *calm* or *peace,* or any other word or phrase that resonates with you.

Best of all, Benson addresses the practice of moving meditation, a tradition within some Eastern faiths, with a strong lineage in Buddhism. He does this in a way that should resonate with any endurance athlete:

> If you are jogging or walking, pay attention to the cadence of your feet on the ground—"left, right, left, right"—and when other thoughts come into your mind, say "Oh, well," and return to "left, right, left, right." Of course, keep your eyes open! Similarly, swimmers can pay attention to the tempo of their strokes, cyclists to the whir of the wheels, dancers to the beat of the music, others to the rhythm of their breathing.[5]

You may have found yourself slipping into this meditative state, which we sometimes call *flow,* at times in your training. In fact, it's often what keeps us coming back to our sports, the sensation of being present with and through the repetitive activity.

Working with a mantra while sitting will make working with a mantra while moving easier, and you'll probably catch yourself using mantra repetition during many of your workouts and races.

Observation Meditation

A more general—and perhaps harder—form of meditation is to simply sit and notice what is happening. Thoughts will arise and subside, and your task is to let them pass through your mind without getting caught up in them. When you find yourself getting tied into the thoughts, you simply notice that engagement, disengage, and return to simple observation.

Such meditation is sometimes likened to watching clouds pass against the sky. But we don't engage with clouds in the same way we do with our thoughts. I've found two physical analogies work really well. At my yoga studio's former location, one of our rooms was directly above a restaurant. During lunch and dinner service, we could hear the voices of the patrons on the floor below. We could tell that people were talking, but we couldn't quite hear what they were saying. If we wanted to bend our ears to the ground, we could probably make out words and sentences, but that would be a lot of work. Instead, we continued with our practice upstairs, recognizing the conversation happening below. Similarly, when I taught in a room with a glass brick wall, I liked to have my students face the wall, which separated the studio from an indoor track. People passed by on the track, at various speeds and sometimes with interesting clothing or gaits. We noticed them through the glass brick, which blurred their images, and we watched them pass by. If we really needed to talk to them, we could go out and catch them, just as we could run downstairs into the restaurant below the studio and grab someone whose voice we recognized. Instead, we cultivate a passive attitude. Without denying the walkers and runners on the track, we notice them, we watch them pass by, and they are gone.

Choosing a Meditation Guide

While meditation doesn't need equipment beyond a timer, it can be useful to follow a guided practice, especially when you are new to mindfulness. This can be an in-person course, an online video, or an app like Headspace or Insight Timer. Don't spend too long trying to choose your guide—jump in and see how you feel during and after. And you don't need to follow a new lesson every time. There's huge value in getting to know one practice intimately and observing the different experiences you have across every session.

YOGA NIDRA AND NON-SLEEP DEEP REST (NSDR)

While the awareness practices just outlined are designed to build your mindfulness moment to moment, another guided approach to meditation can help you relax. Look for recordings that offer yoga nidra—*nidra* means sleep—or Non-Sleep Deep Rest (NSDR) guidance. Similar to hypnotherapy, these practices can be deeply relaxing. They can't do what some teachers claim: substitute for sleep, especially the restorative sleep that happens late in the night. Try a few, though, and you might find they are a sweet lead-in to an afternoon nap or that they work in well as a stand-alone practice for you—especially if you find it hard to keep your attention on one of the simpler techniques outlined earlier.

Visit sagerountree.com/recovery for a free follow-along yoga nidra meditation.

MINDFUL BREATHING

Learning how to breathe and practicing deep diaphragmatic breathing is easy. And once you've learned this skill, it's available to you virtually all the time, whether you're training, meditating, working, or lying down to sleep. These deep breaths stimulate the vagus nerve and help engage the parasympathetic nervous system, engaging the relaxation response, calming you down, and facilitating recovery.

In addition, deep, mindful breathing can have an antioxidant effect. One study shows that purposeful diaphragmatic breathing and concentration on the breath helped decrease cortisol and increase melatonin in athletes, meaning it reduced the oxidative stress exercise puts on the body.[6] Spending some time focusing on your breathing—the athletes in the study spent an hour, but you can do less—will have a direct, positive effect on your recovery. A recent study showed that conscious slow breathing with HRV biofeedback decreased inflammatory cytokines,[7] underscoring the power of the breath for regulating not only the mind but also the whole system.

Sport psychologist Kate Hays teaches diaphragmatic breathing to her athletes "because it ultimately becomes the fastest way that one can regulate the level of arousal, whether to increase or, more often, to decrease one's level of tension. All kinds of things can be attached to it, images, mood words, cognitions." Your breathing practice can thus be part of your mental training. It can also set the mood for meditation, or it can be a stand-alone practice. As with meditation, you can follow these instructions, take an in-person lesson, or use an app or other recording.

The easiest position for learning this deep breathing is lying on your back, so that you can feel the actions of the breath more easily. If your lower back doesn't feel good as you rest with your legs straight, bend your knees. You can also support your legs with a pillow or two taken off the bed. A position like the supported backbend described in chapter 16 is another good choice for breathing awareness, because it opens the ribcage and makes more room for your breath.

From this comfortable reclining position, begin by simply observing how your breath moves in the space of your body. What areas move as you breathe in? In what direction do they move? In what order? And what happens on exhalation? How does exhalation mirror the action of inhalation, and how do they differ?

Now place one hand on your belly, over your navel, and the other on your chest, above your heart. Can you feel action under and on either side of your hands? Observe that movement for a few breaths. Imagine that your abdomen and thorax are divided into three chambers. The first chamber is your belly, beneath your lower hand. As you inhale, your diaphragm drops down, expanding your abdomen and creating negative air pressure that draws air into your lungs. You'll feel the space between your hands—the second chamber—expand as your lungs fill. And at the very top of each inhalation, bring your awareness to the third chamber, the space above your top hand, where your upper chest expands and your collarbone lifts. Paying closer attention, you might feel the action happening in all three areas simultaneously. Physically, of course, air is entering from the top down. Can you feel that? And can you feel, on the other hand, that the action is initiated from the diaphragm? This three-part breath fully engages the muscles of respiration and leads to a very full inhalation. You'll feel a release from each of these areas as you exhale, probably from the top to the bottom, although it could be in a reverse order, bottom to top, or from all three areas simultaneously. Place your hands by your sides and follow this same action.

Imagine yourself lying on the beach. Your breath is a wave that laps over you from the bottom of your belly to the top of your chest as it comes in. As you exhale, the wave recedes from the top to the bottom, and the water settles into the spaces between the grains of sand.

Once you're comfortable with the mechanism of how your breath moves in the space of your body, you can start to play with various breath ratios, changing how the breath moves in your body across time. First, notice what happens at the top of each inhalation, before the exhalation begins. There's a slight pause there, a moment where the breath is neither coming nor going, just as when the wave is lapping on the shore but you can't tell which direction it's moving. Pause here for just a beat and then return to a full exhalation. At the other end of the breath, notice the correlating pause between exhalation and inhalation—a moment like that when the next wave hasn't yet begun its progress to shore. Suspend the breath here, too, and let that brief pause echo the pause you inserted at the top of inhalation. Continue with this pattern: inhale; rest in fullness; exhale; rest in emptiness. After a few rounds, return to a naturally long breath and observe how you feel.

Next, begin to draw out your exhalation. You can do this with or without the brief retention after inhalation and exhalation. Extending the exhalation will stimulate your vagus nerve, helping slow your pulse and calm you down further. Imagine it as an outgoing tide—each exhalation lasts slightly longer than the inhalation that preceded it. You can measure this qualitatively, letting each exhalation *feel* longer than your inhalations, or you can quantify by counting the beats of inhalation and the beats of exhalation and letting the exhalations measure a few beats longer than the inhalations. Continue for a few rounds, then return to a comfortably long breath. Observe how you feel.

You'll find a follow-along audio file with accompanying breathing cues at sagerountree.com/recovery.

Come back to diaphragmatic breathing throughout your day. The more you practice, the more you'll be able to return to this natural, full breath. Breath awareness teaches body awareness, and body awareness is crucial for both your recovery and your success as an athlete. Sport psychology consultant and former professional cyclist Kristin Keim says, "It would benefit more athletes in sleep and recovery if they took more time to properly stretch, breathe, center, and harness their awareness to their body. You can tell a huge difference between pros and amateurs by the level of psychological and physiological awareness they have of their own bodies."

QUICK TIPS

- A few minutes of meditation on most days can improve your recovery and your endurance.
- The goal of meditation is not to stop thinking; it's to become aware of the thinking and to return to focus without getting swept up in thought.
- Deep diaphragmatic breathing can accompany meditation or be a stand-alone practice.

Part III

RECOVERY PROTOCOLS

18

Putting It Together

In this part of the book, we'll integrate the elements from the preceding parts. The following chapters look at recovery routines to target various training and race distances/competitions. Depending on your age, your history with the sport, the effort expended in the event, and the sport itself—specifically, how much running it involves and hence how much impact it places on your legs—your own recovery choices and the amount of time your recovery takes can vary widely.

Remembering that time is the most important recovery tool, let's take a look at factors that contribute to your recovery time. One rule of thumb used for running dictates running easy for X days after your race, where X is the number of miles run. But we can finesse this further (and include other sports beyond running) by basing time to recover on time spent racing. U.S. Olympic triathlon coach Gale Bernhardt estimates that a bike race requires 1–3 days per hour of racing done, a triathlon requires 3–5 days per hour of racing done, and a running race requires 4–6 days per hour of racing done. My experience, and those of my athletes, bears this out, and it's a much more broadly applicable scale than the usual rule of thumb that metes out a day of recovery for each mile run in a race. If you do not race but play a team sport or compete in another discipline, consider the level of impact, from none (bike racing) to lots (running and contact sports) to use these guidelines accordingly.

Bernhardt also created a table weighing the subjective factors that affect time to recover after a race. Working from table 18.1, you can further predict the time until full recovery by seeing how many scores you have in columns 2 and 3. The more you have, the longer you can expect recovery to take. If you wind up injured or sick after the race, that further prolongs your recovery time. Looking at the table, you'll know whether to expect recovery to slide toward the shorter or the longer end of the scale.

Table 18.1 illustrates the importance of managing stress both before and after the race, as well as the importance of nutrition before, during, and after the race. These are factors within your control. Also within your control, with some long-term planning, is your training: the level of

Table 18.1.   Recovery after racing. © *Gale Bernhardt. Adapted with permission*

RANKING VALUE	1	2	3
BEFORE THE RACE			
1. Age	<40	40–60	60+
2. Conditioning	High	Medium	Low
3. Nutritional status	Great	Average	Poor
4. Taper and rest	Great	Average	Poor
5. Athletic experience in the sport	>10 years	5–10 years	<5 years
6. Life stress (family/job/personal/travel)	Low	Medium	High
THE RACE			
1. Sport	Cycling	Triathlon	Running
2. Distance of the event (relative to ability)	Short	Medium	Long
3. Racing intensity (relative to race distance)	Using it as a training day	Medium intensity	All-out, highest average speed
4. Nutritional practice (fueling/hydration)	Great	Average	Poor
5. Course	Easy	Moderate	Difficult
6. Weather conditions (temperature/humidity)	Perfect	Okay	Bad
AFTER THE RACE			
1. Nutritional practice (fueling/hydration)	Great	Average	Poor
2. Life stress (family/job/personal/travel)	Low	Medium	High
3. Workouts following the event (intensity/duration)	Easy/short	Moderate	Fast/long

conditioning you bring to the race, the care you take in your taper, and your effort on race day, which most directly affects recovery time. Wise progression throughout a career will build your athletic experience in the sport and your ability at various distances, as well as your ability to eat and drink and pace yourself correctly during the race. While weather conditions are obviously out of your control come race day, the workouts you do in the week after the event are surely in your control. Don't jettison your recovery by rushing back to training too quickly.

Managing these controllable factors is the sign of a well-balanced athlete. If you can keep your nutrition up, your stress down, and your training progressive and balanced, you're likely to recover well. As physiologist Bill Sands told me, "There is nothing powerful enough in the recovery area to overcome stupid coaching, bad planning, and no talent. Periodize properly, train intelligently, eat right, and have a smart coach." Once you have these lifestyle elements in balance, you can focus on the other recovery techniques covered in part II of this book to enhance your recovery. In the final chapters of this book, we'll see how these techniques might fit into a time line.

Your recovery is relative to your experience. Jamie Donaldson, first female and third overall at the 2010 Badwater ultramarathon, remembers: "When I first started ultras, it took me months to recover. For example, when I did the Badwater ultramarathon in 2007, I couldn't even run for a month afterward. In 2009, I completed Badwater and was able to run competitively in the Leadville Trail 100 mile less than three weeks later. The training you put in ahead of time is almost as important to your recovery as to what you do after the race." Your body will respond to the demands of the event relative to your past experience, whether you ever achieve elite status like Donaldson's.

Gordo Byrn, endurance coach and coauthor of *Going Long*, agrees. "Recovery after races is really individual," he says. "Someone under a lot of life stress might take six months to recover from a half-Ironman, while an elite athlete might be back to relatively normal training in four or five days."

The more your body is conditioned to the demands of your sport and the more times you go through the routines of recovery, the quicker your body will adapt and respond and the sooner you will be ready to resume training—to a point. As you age, you'll need to take care to follow your body's cues. What worked five years ago might not be enough now; recovery times will lengthen as you age.

ELEMENTS TO INCLUDE YEAR-ROUND

Beyond the time you spend following the protocols listed in the next two chapters, here are some elements that will aid your recovery and your training, along with a suggestion of frequency. Choose the elements that apply to you and that you can keep up with regularly.

Daily

Take a moment to note how you feel qualitatively.

Log your workouts and recovery metrics.

Make a point to spend time focusing on elements besides training.

Nap and/or focus on getting enough nightly sleep.

Eat a healthy, varied diet.

Take an omega-3 supplement, about 1,000 mg of EHA/DHA combined, or 1 tablespoon flaxseed, or 1 teaspoon flaxseed oil.

Draw a warm bath.

Make time for meditation and/or restorative yoga poses, especially legs up the wall.

Weekly

Check in with your log, realigning with your goals and assessing overall stress level. Tweak as needed.

After hard workouts, put on recovery socks and use compression sleeves, if you have access to them.

Spend 15 minutes or so in the sauna after your workouts a few days each week.

Sit in the whirlpool briefly; space your visit far apart from hard workouts.

Perform self-massage 3–4 times a week.

Schedule a massage with a licensed massage therapist weekly or bi-weekly, depending on needs and budget.

Do a longer, restorative yoga session 2–3 times a week at home or at a studio.

Monthly

Meet with a sports psychologist to discuss your goals and mental skills.

Meet with a sports dietitian to discuss your nutrition.

Quarterly

Check that your running shoes are in good shape; if not, replace them.

Biannually

Assess your bike fit and equipment, especially if you have changed elements of your training.

Have your technique analyzed by a coach, especially in swimming.

Annually

Get a complete physical, ideally from a health care provider familiar with athletes.

RECOVERY BETWEEN SEASONS

The chapters that follow show what to do in the few hours and days after a tough workout or competition. Beyond that, you must allot even more time for deep physical and mental recovery after your peak race of the season. If you are always turning around and moving straight into the next cycle, you will never achieve long-term recovery, and eventually you will shortchange your performance.

Take at least one week, possibly two together, after your peak event of the year. (Better still, have two transition weeks, one after your spring peak and one after your fall peak.) During this transition time, break out of your usual habits. You might choose to try a different sport or only to walk. Recharging your batteries, both physiologically and psychologically, will ensure that you continue to enjoy your training in the next cycle and that you come to your next cycle with the appropriate mental and physical resources.

Create as much distance from routine as you can in this transition period. It might coincide with a vacation—a chance to spend more time with your family and friends—or you might simply keep your bike packed in its travel box or propped in the garage, your running shoes hung to dry.

Here are some cues from ultrarunners, whose peak events are run on a grand scale and thus demand a grand attention to recovery. Kami Semick told me, "Since the ultra season is so long, I take an annual break away from running. During this break period, I will take a few days of complete rest (typically after my last race of the season), then for three or four weeks, I will primarily ski for fun (Nordic and downhill), and pool run. For a total of four to six weeks, I will not do any quality running efforts and I will keep my runs below two hours."

This restoration happens not simply on the physical level. Consider the psychological elements of recovery between long events, too. Ultrarunner Annette Bednosky, women's winner at the 2010 Burning River 100 Mile Endurance Run, says, "Recovering from a focus race is about taking time off mentally as much as physically. For instance, [in early 2010] right after Mad City, I did jump right into an ice bath for a 15-minute soak accompanied by a glass of wine and then a nap. For the next week, I tried not to think about running, racing, or future training. I exercised each day—doing different things—yet it was important not to have any sort of performance or training focus."

Former *Runner's World* editor Jennifer Van Allen agrees, and she underscores the point that you must be in tune with your goals and your body so you can give yourself what you need, rather than following a prescribed formula to determine when you will be recovered. "I never quite follow the mile-per-day rule; I listen to my body and figure out what I need," she says. "After I run a race, I'm so excited, my love for running is at its height; it's the time when I want to run the most, and my body will not cooperate. It's tough for me to hold back. I have to coach myself to not get out there, because that's when I'm most fragile." Van Allen learned this from experience, when she ran four marathons in four consecutive weeks in fall 2009. "The morning after the Richmond Marathon, I wanted to get moving," she remembers. "I went out, and I was so enjoying my run in downtown Richmond but I wasn't moving really well. My gait was sloppy. I tripped over cobblestones and cut my face and elbows. That's a small example of the danger of doing more than I was ready for."

How long should this interseason recovery period last? Here's an easy rule: Look at the number of hours you trained in your peak week of volume, and take that many days free of structured training objectives. If you maxed out at 7 hours a week, an easy week without formal workouts should suffice. If you regularly train 20 hours a week, though, you will do well to take a full three weeks' mental break.

As with everything, however, your recovery time depends on your history and goals. A week or two might do after a shorter event; it might take a month or more to regain interest in training after a longer race. Consider all the stories of people who don't ride again for months following an Ironman (my own story among them—I transitioned from the Ironman into a distance-running block that included the New York Marathon and a 50K, and my bike hung unused on the garage wall). This is not a training failure, as long as you have a reasonable race schedule that won't have you out again too soon, and provided that you are staying active in other sports. It's evidence that you're listening to your body's needs and training because you feel passionate about it. When that is your guiding principle, you'll have balance in your life, and training will enhance your experience—not dominate it.

19

Recovery from Short-Distance Training and Racing

The most practical recovery technique for you will be the one that you actually *do*. Hence, as you consider these recovery protocols, think about what works well for you. What have you found worth your time and money? Are you good at self-massage, or is it worth paying a massage therapist? Do you swear by ice baths? Would you never travel without your compression socks, or are you a minimalist? Select from the elements of the protocols laid out here to devise a plan that will work for you. I offer both a full-featured version and a fast-fix version.

How you define "short" depends on your individual history. For the purposes of this chapter, we'll call short races those lasting under two hours, or, for experienced competitors, as long as a two-hour-plus Olympic distance triathlon. For many training sessions for short events, special attention to a recovery protocol isn't necessary. You'll want to ensure you are getting enough sleep, eating a variety of healthy foods, and managing your overall stress load. Proper attention to these three elements will do wonders for your recovery, for your training, and for your life.

During the course of training for a short-course event, however, you'll have some workouts that should prompt more specific attention to recovery. After workouts that are very intense or on the longer side, you'll want to be sure you've devoted some attention to setting up your recovery. Intensity varies from person to person, but an intense workout is one intended to push your limits, either in speed or in distance or duration. For recovery purposes, we can define longer workouts as those that last 90 minutes or longer and/or take 15 minutes longer than your most recent long workout.

After your peak event of the training cycle, the focus you give to recovery will help set up your next training cycle. Be careful to give your body the care and time it needs after the race before you start the next block.

RECOVERY PROTOCOL DURING SHORT-DISTANCE TRAINING

Your recovery begins before the end of your workout, in your cooldown (see table 19.1). Let this be 10 or more minutes of easy, light activity. It can grow progressively easier, so that you are finishing a run with a walk, a ride with a really easy spin, or a swim with some floating and light kicking. Once you stop moving, gently stretch the muscle groups you used in the workout. Don't push deeply; do take advantage of your increased blood flow to elongate the muscle fibers and prevent the formation of muscular adhesions. As you stretch, sip on a sports drink to rehydrate and take in some calories.

After your stretch but before you shower, if you find any areas feel especially sore or tender, you can spot-ice them for 10 minutes or so. As you do, reflect on why that area feels sore. Could your biomechanics be improved?

While you ice or after you stretch, take in a recovery snack with plenty of carbohydrates and continue hydrating. Then get clean and resume your regular good nutrition habits, eating a variety of fruits, vegetables, whole grains, lean proteins, and healthy fats.

As you go through the day, you might slot in a massage or simply wear recovery garments. Yoga and/or meditation can also help you relax and boost your recovery. At some point, either nap or simply take a few minutes to put your feet up. Toward the end of the afternoon, a little light activity will get your blood moving and diminish soreness. Take

Table 19.1. Recovery protocol during short-distance training

TIME AFTER FINISHING WORKOUT	ACTIVITY
-00:10	Cool down, 10 minutes
00:00	Stretch, rehydrate
00:15	Spot-ice any areas that need attention
00:30	Snack
00:40	Shower
1:00	Massage, 1 hour
2:00	Don recovery garments
2:30	Meal
3:00	Yoga/breathing/meditation
3:30	Nap, 40 minutes
4:15	Walk
5:00	Self-massage with foam roller
10:00–12:00	Warm bath before bedtime
1 day	Lighter workout, possibly in another sport

your dog or a neighbor's for a walk around the block or go on a short hike with your friends or kids. Afterward, you might make a few passes over your muscles with a foam roller.

Be sure to get to bed early enough to ensure you have plenty of sleep. As part of your bedtime routine, soak in a warm bath, adding Epsom salts if you like.

In the next day or two, keep an eye on your recovery from the workout. Take care that you don't work too hard, especially in the same sport, the day following an intense or long workout.

RECOVERY PROTOCOL AFTER SHORT-DISTANCE RACING

After a race, you can follow the same general protocol you've developed during training, but pay special attention to refueling, rehydrating, resting, and resuming training gradually (see table 19.2). Begin with 10 minutes of walking to stabilize your heart rate and blood pressure.

When you are at a race, instead of merely finishing a workout at your house, it can be harder to secure a proper recovery snack. Think ahead and pack your own, or make good choices among the postrace offerings. Look for carbs and lean protein and be sure you include some sodium to aid your rehydration efforts. Keep sipping on water or a sports drink through the hours after the race.

Check that your body temperature is stable. If conditions are very hot, cool down by sitting in a lake or kiddie pool (once the drinks are gone) or by dousing yourself with water. If it is cold out, change into warm, dry clothes.

If massages are offered, get one, but do communicate with the therapist. This is the time for a light flush-out, not deep tissue work. Afterward, put on your compression socks or tights.

Spend some time reflecting and processing your experience. This can be journaling, chatting with training or life partners, or talking to a coach or a sport psychologist.

Do get off your feet and rest, but intersperse such rest with bouts of movement. If you're traveling home some distance in the car, be sure to stop periodically and walk around. (If you're rehydrating properly, you'll need a pit stop every hour or two.)

In the day after your race, a brief (30-minute) recovery workout will help relieve soreness. Depending on your sport, this could be a walk, a spin on the bike, or a light swim. Don't run. Delayed-onset muscle soreness (DOMS) usually peaks in the second day after the event, when a day of total rest is usually in order. It's a good time to write your race report, now that you've had some time to process and reflect. This will help you put your experience into context. Expect to have changing

Table 19.2. Recovery protocol after short-distance racing

TIME AFTER FINISHING RACE	ACTIVITY
-10:00	Cool down, 10 minutes
00:00	Stretch, rehydrate
00:15	Snack
00:30	Cool off/warm up
00:45	Massage
1:30	Processing: Talk about your experience with your coach or a buddy, or journal (this can be a race report or something more individual and private)
1:45	Shower
2:00	Don recovery garments
2:30	Meal
3:00	Yoga/breathing/meditation
3:30	Nap, 40 minutes to 2 hours
4:15–6:00	Walk 20–30 minutes
10:00–12:00	Warm bath before bedtime
1 day	Walk/spin/swim
2 days	Rest

emotions no matter how you did; it's common to cycle through a range of feelings, good and bad, and expecting them is part of the process.

A massage on the third day will help set you up for your next training cycle. Return to training carefully, paying attention to indicators of your recovery. Don't confuse poor performance in training after the race as a loss of fitness. Often, it's a sign that more recovery is in order.

20

Recovery from Long-Distance Training and Racing

Longer workouts require a longer recovery and more attention to the signs of your recovery so that you don't layer on another hard workout too soon. The more you value your performance in distance events, the more you'll need to emphasize your recovery.

Be sure that the workout is bookended by easier activity, both in daily life and in your preceding and subsequent training sessions, unless you are consciously choosing to stack long workouts together back to back—in which case, recovery becomes even more crucial.

RECOVERY PROTOCOL DURING LONG-DISTANCE TRAINING
The recovery periods following long-distance workouts are training for your recovery postrace. Follow a consistent protocol once you have determined the elements that work best for you. It might look something like this (see table 20.1): Start with a cooldown and a very light stretch, accompanied with a drink to rehydrate. After a workout with 90 minutes to 2 hours of running, consider spending 10 to 15 minutes in a cool or ice bath. You can eat a warm recovery snack as you do. (If there was no running involved but something feels a little tweaked, spot-ice and consider what changed to incur that tweaky feeling.)

After your shower, or later in the afternoon, a massage can be a useful part of your routine. Be sure to tell your therapist how you're feel-

Table 20.1. Recovery protocol during long-distance training

TIME AFTER FINISHING RACE	ACTIVITY
-00:10	Cool down, 10 minutes
00:00	Stretch, rehydrate
00:30	Snack
00:40	Shower
1:00	Massage, 1 hour
2:00	Don recovery garments/ peristaltic compression
2:30	Meal
3:00	Yoga/breathing/meditation
3:30	Nap, 40 minutes
4:15	Walk
5:00	Self-massage with foam roller
10:00–12:00	Warm bath before bedtime
1 day	Lighter workout, possibly in another sport

ing and that you've had a long workout. If you like compression socks or tights, add them after your shower or massage. They can come off before your nap—or stay on. If you have access to a NormaTec MVP machine, by all means, use it!

Throughout the day, eat well. Take in some protein and continue rehydrating. In the afternoon, some light yoga, breathing exercises, or meditation can help. (When you've just eaten, be very gentle with your yoga.) This quiet time can set you up for a nap, or you can simply put your feet up and read or rest quietly.

Before dinner, take a walk around the block, followed by a short massage with a foam roller (it won't be necessary if you've had a massage earlier in the day). Then eat well, choose a relaxing activity, and move through a restful bedtime routine that might include a warm bath.

Be sure to follow your longer workout days with easier days consisting of a lighter workout, possibly in another sport. Take care that the intensity is not too high.

RECOVERY PROTOCOL AFTER LONG-DISTANCE RACING

The protocol to follow after your peak distance events adds to what you've established in training (see table 20.2). You'll need to adjust your

Table 20.2. Recovery protocol after long-distance racing

TIME AFTER FINISHING RACE	ACTIVITY
00:00	Walk
00:05	Rehydrate
00:15	Snack
00:30	Cool off/warm up
00:45	Massage
1:45	Shower
2:00	Don recovery garments/ peristaltic compression; work on processing your experience by talking to your coach or a friend, or by writing
2:30	Meal
3:00	Yoga/breathing/meditation
3:30	Nap, 40 minutes to 2 hours
4:15–6:00	Walk 10–20 minutes
10:00–12:00	Warm bath before bedtime
1 day	Walk or float
2 days	Rest
3 days	Walk or float
1 day–14 days	Replenish

routine based on location. For example, if you've raced a triathlon in a cool lake, you might enjoy your snack sitting waist-deep in the water. Alternatively, if you are racing in cold conditions, change into warm clothes. You might choose a massage at the race site, but make sure it's very light. Continue with the afternoon and evening recovery routine you've established, mixing in some time for celebration.

In the days following your event, moving around is very important; workouts are not. The day after the race, enjoy a short, slow walk, or float in a warm (not hot) pool. Delayed-onset muscle soreness (DOMS) usually peaks in the second day after the event, when a day of total rest is usually in order. It's a good time to write your race report, now that you've had some time to process and reflect. As sports psychologist Danielle Adams Norenberg suggests, this is the time to allow the emotions to come and go while you stay present and focus on connecting with your friends and family. In the days and weeks following your event, be sure to eat plenty of high-quality food, to rehydrate, to sleep, and to take the time for mental restoration.

Recovery between Back-to-Back Races

Back-to-back events require special attention to recovery. They include running legs of a relay race covering 200 miles or more, such as Hood to Coast, or being part of a mountain bike race team. Cycling races have long included weekends and weeks offering more than one race. With the growing popularity of multisport, race directors are staging more than one race at a venue in the same weekend. Here in North Carolina, "doing a double" — racing both races — is a popular (and macho) thing to do. Physiologically, the two races blend together into one single event, so you can project your time to recovery by adding together the two.

My athlete Katy did the double at White Lake, North Carolina, in 2010, racing the half-iron-distance race on Saturday and the sprint triathlon on Sunday. She followed the protocol outlined in tables 20.1 and 20.2, to good effect.

Here is what I suggested to her in the week before the race, with my notes in square brackets:

You know what to do this week and during the race. Be smart and happy and it'll be all good. But here's what I want you to do AFTER the half so that you can make it through the sprint also feeling happy. Timing is important:

1. As SOON as you finish, regardless of hunger, eat/drink 200–300 calories, mostly carbs, with some protein as you've been practicing. Recovery drink, or a smoothie, or a bagel and peanut butter. I can't stress this enough. [Protein works well for Katy.]

2. Go home. Get showered. Get on cozy clothes. If you have recovery socks (I think you do, yes? White ones?), put them on.

3. Eat a good meal. Again, protein. Gatorade or similar. Rehydrate, rehydrate, rehydrate. This meal should be within two hours of the finish.

4. Advil if you need it. [While you shouldn't rely on long-term use of NSAIDs nor use them during the event, in a situation like this, they can help reduce inflammation in the short term and alleviate pain so the nap goes better.]

5. Lie down, prop your feet up, and nap if you can.

6. Around dinnertime, do some light walking.

7. One beer, good; two beers, better; three beers, uh-oh. (Beer can read "glass of wine.") [The goal here is to support the fun of the race weekend.]

8. Sleep.

9. Sunday morning, don't worry if you start out stiff. You will probably be surprised at how the swim loosens you up.

It was very hot on race day for the half-iron-distance. Temperatures reached the 90s, and the run course has very little shade. Katy struggled but made it, and she did very well in the sprint, finishing very happy and satisfied. She added this postscript to her race report, sent to her triathlon club:

There were several things I did directly after the half-iron that I think were KEY! I immediately consumed about 200 calories, then I sat in the very cold lake for a good long time. Then I cleaned up, went back to the hotel and ate a huge turkey sandwich on whole wheat with a bunch of Doritos. Doritos suck, but they are loaded with salt and I think I really needed that. I also drank about a half gallon of water and then took a good nap (instead of watching the Kentucky Derby).

EYES ON THE PRIZE

In the yoga classes I teach, we begin by setting an intention for the practice, and at the end, we realign with that original intention before recommitting to it or revising it into something that will work off the mat. When I prescribe workouts for my athletes, I make sure it's very clear why we're doing them—how they serve the bigger plan and the athlete's goals. Do the same for your own training and recovery practices. Throughout your career, keep your eyes on the big picture.

Is your goal to reach a personal record at one big race each year? Recovery is crucial to your proper peaking. Is it to compete well across a series of races or a season of games? Recovery will help you string together more than one strong showing. Is it to have your training and competition be a healthy and balanced part of your life? Recovery will ensure that you keep your perspective.

Just as it's more rewarding to climb into bed after a productive day, your recovery will be more fulfilling when it serves to balance the work you do. Keep the ratio of stress and rest in your favor by prioritizing your recovery, and your sport will be a valued, fruitful part of your life for years to come.

Notes

CHAPTER 1. WHY RECOVERY MATTERS

1. N. D. Gill, C. M. Beaven, and C. Cook, "Effectiveness of Post-match Recovery Strategies in Rugby Players," *British Journal of Sports Medicine* 40 (2006): 260–63.

2. T. O. Bompa and G. G. Haff, *Periodization*, 5th ed. (Champaign, IL: Human Kinetics, 2009).

3. Joe Friel, *The Triathlete's Training Bible*, 3rd ed. (Boulder, CO: Velo, 2009).

CHAPTER 3. QUALITATIVE MEASUREMENTS OF RECOVERY

1. D. McNair, M. Lorr, and L. F. Droppleman, *Profile of Mood States Manual* (San Diego: Educational and Industrial Testing Service, 1971, 1992).

2. Michael Kellmann and K. Wolfgang Kallus, *Recovery-Stress Questionnaire for Athletes: User Manual* (Champaign, IL: Human Kinetics, 2001).

3. S. L. Gnacinski, B. B. Meyer, and C. A. Wahl, "Psychometric Properties of the RESTQ-Sport-36 in a Collegiate Student-Athlete Population," *Frontiers in Psychology* 12 (2021), https://doi.org/10.3389/fpsyg.2021.671919 (20 March 2023).

4. Michael Kellmann, Tom Patrick, Cal Botterill, and Clare Wilson, "The Recovery-Cue and Its Use in Applied Settings: Practical Suggestions

Regarding Assessment and Monitoring of Recovery," in *Enhancing Recovery: Preventing Underperformance in Athletes*, ed. M. Kellmann (Champaign, IL: Human Kinetics, 2002), 219–29.

5. Kellmann, Patrick, Botterill, and Wilson, "The Recovery-Cue and Its Use in Applied Settings," n.p.

6. Matt Fitzgerald, *Run: The Mind-Body Method of Running by Feel* (Boulder, CO: Velo, 2010).

CHAPTER 4. QUANTITATIVE MEASUREMENTS OF RECOVERY

1. A. C. Snyder et al., "A Physiological/Psychological Indicator of Over-Reaching during Intensive Training," *International Journal of Sports Medicine* 14 (1993): 29–32.

2. Carl Foster, "Monitoring Training in Athletes with Reference to Overtraining Syndrome," *Medicine and Science in Sports and Exercise* 30 (1998): 1164–68.

CHAPTER 5. RECOVERY FROM INJURY AND ILLNESS

1. Here's an example of guidelines at the time of publication: M. G. Wilson et al., "Cardiorespiratory Considerations for Return-to-Play in Elite Athletes after COVID-19 Infection: A Practical Guide for Sport and Exercise Medicine Physicians," *British Journal of Sports Medicine* 54 (2020): 1157–61, https://bjsm.bmj.com/content/54/19/1157 (4 March 2023).

CHAPTER 6. ACTIVE RECOVERY

1. F. B. Neric et al., "Comparison of Swim Recovery and Muscle Stimulation on Lactate Removal after Sprint Swimming," *Journal of Strength and Conditioning Research* 23 (2009): 2560–67.

2. I. Wigernaes et al., "Active Recovery Reduces the Decrease in Circulating White Blood Cells after Exercise," *International Journal of Sports Medicine* 21 (2000): 608–12.

3. C. Baldari et al., "Blood Lactate Removal during Recovery at Various Intensities Below the Individual Anaerobic Threshold in Triathletes," *Journal of Sports Medicine and Physical Fitness* 45 (2005): 460–66.

CHAPTER 7. STRESS REDUCTION

1. M. A. Stults-Kolehmainen and J. B. Bartholomew, "Psychological Stress Impairs Short-Term Muscular Recovery from Resistance Exercise," *Medicine and Science in Sports and Exercise* 44, no. 11 (2012): 2220–27, https://doi.org/10.1249/MSS.0b013e31825f67a0 (4 March 2023).

CHAPTER 8. SLEEP

1. C. D. Mah et al., "The Effects of Sleep Extension on the Athletic Performance of Collegiate Basketball Players," *Sleep* 34, no. 7 (2011): 943–50, https://doi.org/10.5665/SLEEP.1132 (4 March 2023).

2. K. Spiegel, R. Leproult, and E. Van Cauter, "Impact of Sleep Debt on Metabolic and Endocrine Function," *Lancet* 354 (1999): 1435–39.

3. A. E. Mesas et al., "Is Daytime Napping an Effective Strategy to Improve Sport-Related Cognitive and Physical Performance and Reduce Fatigue? A Systematic Review and Meta-analysis of Randomised Controlled Trials," *British Journal of Sports Medicine* online, 23 January 2023, https://bjsm.bmj.com/content/early/2023/01/22/bjsports-2022-106355 (4 March 2023).

4. See, for example, M. W. Driller et al., "Pyjamas, Polysomnography, and Professional Athletes: The Role of Sleep Tracking Technology in Sport," *Sports* 11, no. 1 (2023): 14, https://doi.org/10.3390/sports11010014 (4 March 2023).

5. C. Draganich and K. Erdal, "Placebo Sleep Affects Cognitive Functioning," *Journal of Experimental Psychology: Learning, Memory, and Cognition* 40, no. 3 (2014): 857–64, https://doi.org/10.1037/a0035546 (4 March 2023); Shadab A. Rahman et al., "Manipulating Sleep Duration Perception Changes Cognitive Performance: An Exploratory Analysis," *Journal of Psychosomatic Research* 132 (2020), https://doi.org/10.1016/j.jpsychores.2020.109992 (4 March 2023).

6. Dimitri Gavriloff et al., "Sham Sleep Feedback Delivered via Actigraphy Biases Daytime Symptom Reports in People with Insomnia: Implications for Insomnia Disorder and Wearable Devices," *Journal of Sleep Research* 27, no. 6 (2018): e12726, https://onlinelibrary.wiley.com/doi/abs/10.1111/jsr.12726 (4 March 2023).

7. Viviana Greco et al., "Wearing an Eye Mask during Overnight Sleep Improves Episodic Learning and Alertness," *Sleep* (2022), doi.org/10.1093 /sleep/zsac305 (4 March 2023).

CHAPTER 9. NUTRITION AND HYDRATION

1. Michael Pollan, *In Defense of Food* (New York: Penguin, 2008), 1.

2. C. M. S. Kerksick et al., "International Society of Sports Nutrition Position Stand: Nutrient Timing," *Journal of the International Society of Sports Nutrition* 14, no. 1 (2017), https://doi.org/10.1186/s12970-017-0189-4 (4 March 2023).

3. J. L. Ivy et al., "Muscle Glycogen Synthesis after Exercise: Effect of Time of Carbohydrate Ingestion," *Journal of Applied Physiology* 64 (1988): 1480–85.

4. J. R. Karp et al., "Chocolate Milk as a Post-exercise Recovery Aid," *International Journal of Sport Nutrition and Exercise Metabolism* 16 (2006): 78–91.

5. Melinda L. Ray et al., "Effect of Sodium in a Rehydration Beverage When Consumed as a Fluid or Meal," *Journal of Applied Physiology* 85, no. 4 (1998): 1329–36, https://doi.org/10.1152/jappl.1998.85.4.1329 (4 March 2023).

CHAPTER 10. SUPPLEMENTS

1. Nicholas B. Tiller, *The Skeptic's Guide to Sports Science: Confronting Myths of the Health and Fitness Industry* (New York: Routledge, 2020).

2. O. S. Neubauer et al., "Antioxidant Responses to an Acute Ultra-endurance Exercise: Impact on DNA Stability and Indications for an Increased Need for Nutritive Antioxidants in the Early Recovery Phase," *British Journal of Nutrition* 104 (2010): 1129–38.

3. Travis Thomas, Kelly Anne Erdman, and Louise M. Burke, "Position of the Academy of Nutrition and Dietetics, Dietitians of Canada, and the American College of Sports Medicine: Nutrition and Athletic Performance," *Academy Position Paper* 116, no. 3 (2016): 501–28, https://doi.org/10.1016/j.jand.2015.12.006 (5 March 2023).

4. M. Negro et al., "Branched-Chain Amino Acid Supplementation Does Not Enhance Athletic Performance but Affects Muscle Recovery and the Immune System," *Journal of Sports Medicine and Physical Fitness* 48 (2008): 347–51.

5. D. G. Rowbottom, D. Keast, and A. R. Morton, "The Emerging Role of Glutamine as an Indicator of Exercise Stress and Overtraining," *Sports Medicine* 21, no. 2 (1996): 80–97.

6. See, for example, H. J. Engels, M. M. Fahlman, and J. C. Wirth, "Effects of Ginseng on Secretory IgA, Performance, and Recovery from Interval Exercise," *Medicine and Science in Sports and Exercise* 35 (2003): 690–96.

CHAPTER 11. COLD AND HEAT

1. Robert D. Hyldahl and Jonathan M. Peake, "Combining Cooling or Heating Applications with Exercise Training to Enhance Performance and Muscle Adaptations," *Journal of Applied Physiology* 129, no. 2 (2020): 353–65.

2. J. R. Broatch, A. Petersen, and D. J. Bishop, "Postexercise Cold Water Immersion Benefits Are Not Greater Than the Placebo Effect," *Medicine and Science in Sports and Exercise* 46, no. 11 (2014): 2139–47, doi.org/10.1249/MSS.0000000000000348 (4 March 2023).

3. Broatch, Petersen, and Bishop, "Postexercise Cold Water Immersion Benefits."

4. P. Angelopoulos et al., "Cold-Water Immersion and Sports Massage Can Improve Pain Sensation but Not Functionality in Athletes with Delayed Onset Muscle Soreness," *Healthcare* (Basel, Switzerland) 10, no. 12 (2022), https://doi.org/10.3390/healthcare10122449 (4 March 2023).

5. Malte Krueger et al., "Whole-Body Cryotherapy (−110 °C) Following High-Intensity Intermittent Exercise Does Not Alter Hormonal, Inflammatory, or

Muscle Damage Biomarkers in Trained Males," *Cytokine* 113 (2019): 277–84, https://doi.org/10.1016/j.cyto.2018.07.018 (4 March 2023).

6. N. V. Kirby et al., "Intermittent Post-exercise Sauna Bathing Improves Markers of Exercise Capacity in Hot and Temperate Conditions in Trained Middle-Distance Runners," *European Journal of Applied Physiology* 121 (2021): 621–35, https://doi.org/10.1007/s00421-020-04541-z (4 March 2023); Guy S. M. Scoon et al., "Effect of Post-exercise Sauna Bathing on the Endurance Performance of Competitive Male Runners," *Journal of Science and Medicine in Sport* 10, no. 4 (2007): 259–62, https://doi.org/10.1016/j.jsams.2006.06.009 (4 March 2023).

7. A. Mero et al., "Effects of Far-Infrared Sauna Bathing on Recovery from Strength and Endurance Training Sessions in Men," *SpringerPlus* 4 (2015), https://doi.org/10.1186/s40064-015-1093-5 (4 March 2023).

8. K. Kauppinen, "Sauna, Shower, and Ice Water Immersion: Physiological Responses to Brief Exposures to Heat, Cool, and Cold, Part I: Body Fluid Balance," *Arctic Medical Research* 48 (1989): 55–63.

CHAPTER 12. HOME TECHNOLOGICAL AIDS
1. D. Lawrence and V. V. Kakkar, "Graduated, Static, External Compression of the Lower Limb: A Physiological Assessment," *British Journal of Surgery* 67 (1980): 119–21.

2. A. Ali, M. P. Caine, and B. G. Snow, "Graduated Compression Stockings: Physiological and Perceptual Responses during and after Exercise," *Journal of Sports Sciences* 25 (2007): 413–19.

3. Elmarie Terblanche and Marlize Coetzee, "The Effect of Graded Compression Socks on Maximal Exercise Capacity and Recovery in Runners," *Medicine and Science in Sports and Exercise* 39, no. 5 (2007): S350, https://doi.org/10.1249/01.mss.0000274369.11864.4b (5 March 2023).

4. V. Davies, K. G. Thompson, and S.-M. Cooper. "The Effects of Compression Garments on Recovery." *Journal of Strength and Conditioning Research* 23 (2009): 1786–94.

5. S. A. Armstrong et al., "Compression Socks and Functional Recovery Following Marathon Running: A Randomized Controlled Trial," *Journal of Strength and Conditioning Research* 29, no. 2 (2015): 528–33, https://doi.org/10.1519/JSC.0000000000000649 (4 March 2023).

6. For one overview, see J. F. Burr et al., "Cannabis and Athletic Performance," *Sports Medicine* 51, suppl. 1 (2021): 75–87, https://doi.org/10.1007/s40279-021-01505-x (4 March 2023).

7. Here's a thorough debunking: Paul Ingraham, "Does Epsom Salt Work? The Science and Mythology of Epsom Salt Bathing for Recovery from Muscle Pain, Soreness, or Injury," *Pain Science* online, 25 December 2021, https://www.painscience.com/articles/epsom-salts.php (5 March 2023).

CHAPTER 13. OTHER TECHNOLOGICAL AIDS

1. Peter Struijs and Gino Kerkhoffs, "Ankle Sprain," *British Medical Journal of Clinical Evidence* 13 (2010): 1115.

2. L. D. Wilkin et al., "Influence of Therapeutic Ultrasound on Skeletal Muscle Regeneration Following Blunt Contusion," *International Journal of Sports Medicine* 25 (2004): 73–77.

3. A. Grunovas et al., "Peripheral and Systemic Circulation after Local Dynamic Exercise and Recovery Using Passive Foot Movement and Electrostimulation," *Journal of Sports Medicine and Physical Fitness* 47 (2007): 335–43.

4. A. Tessitore et al., "Effectiveness of Active versus Passive Recovery Strategies after Futsal Games," *Journal of Strength and Conditioning Research* 22 (2008): 1402–12.

5. Vipan Broderick, Liis Uiga, and Matthew Driller, "Flotation-Restricted Environmental Stimulation Therapy Improves Sleep and Performance Recovery in Athletes," *Performance Enhancement and Health*, 7, no. 1–2 (2019), https://doi.org/10.1016/j.peh.2019.100149 (4 March 2023).

6. M. R. Hamblin, "Mechanisms and Mitochondrial Redox Signaling in Photobiomodulation," *Photochemistry and Photobiology* 94, no. 2 (2018): 199–212, https://doi.org/10.1111/php.12864 (4 March 2023).

7. D. Barber et al., "Halotherapy for Chronic Respiratory Disorders: From the Cave to the Clinical," *Alternative Therapies in Health and Medicine* 28, no. 3 (2022): 52–56, https://pubmed.ncbi.nlm.nih.gov/32827399/ (4 March 2023).

CHAPTER 14. MASSAGE

1. P. Weerapong, P. A. Hume, and G. S. Kolt, "The Mechanisms of Massage and Effects on Performance, Muscle Recovery, and Injury Prevention," *Sports Medicine* 35 (2005): 235–56.

2. For a meta-analysis, see W. Poppendieck et al., "Massage and Performance Recovery: A Meta-analytical Review," *Sports Medicine* 46 (2016): 183–204, https://doi.org/10.1007/s40279-015-0420-x (5 March 2023).

3. C. A. Mancinelli et al., "The Effects of Massage on Delayed Onset Muscle Soreness and Physical Performance in Female Collegiate Athletes," *Physical Therapy in Sport* 7 (2006): 5–13.

4. Anthony Barnett, "Using Recovery Modalities between Training Sessions in Elite Athletes: Does It Help?" *Sports Medicine* 36 (2006): 781–96.

5. T. M. Best et al., "Effectiveness of Sports Massage for Recovery of Skeletal Muscle from Strenuous Exercise," *Clinical Journal of Sports Medicine* 18 (2008): 446–60.

6. E. V. Wiltshire et al., "Massage Impairs Postexercise Muscle Blood Flow and 'Lactic Acid' Removal." *Medicine and Science in Sports and Exercise* 42 (2010): 1062–71.

7. Pat Archer, *Therapeutic Massage in Athletics* (Baltimore: Lippincott, Williams, and Wilkins, 2007).

8. B. Hemmings et al., "Effects of Massage on Physiological Restoration, Perceived Recovery, and Repeated Sports Performance," *British Journal of Sports Medicine* 34 (2000): 113.

9. José Afonso et al., "The Effectiveness of Post-exercise Stretching in Short-Term and Delayed Recovery of Strength, Range of Motion and Delayed Onset Muscle Soreness: A Systematic Review and Meta-analysis of Randomized

Controlled Trials," *Frontiers in Physiology* 12 (2021), https://doi.org/10.3389/fphys.2021.677581 (5 March 2023).

CHAPTER 15. SELF-MASSAGE

1. R. M. Ferreira, P. N. Martins, and R. S. Goncalves, "Effects of Self-Myofascial Release Instruments on Performance and Recovery: An Umbrella Review," *International Journal of Exercise Science* 15, no. 3 (2022): 861–83, https://www.ncbi.nlm.nih.gov/pmc/articles/PMC9362891/ (5 March 2023).

2. Graham MacDonald et al., "Foam Rolling as a Recovery Tool After an Intense Bout of Physical Activity," *Medicine and Science in Sports and Exercise* 46, no. 1 (2014): 131–42, https://journals.lww.com/acsm-msse/Fulltext/2014/01000/Foam_Rolling_as_a_Recovery_Tool_after_an_Intense.19.aspx (5 March 2023).

3. T. Wiewelhove et al., "A Meta-analysis of the Effects of Foam Rolling on Performance and Recovery," *Frontiers in Physiology* 10 (2019): 376, https://doi.org/10.3389/fphys.2019.00376 (5 March 2023).

4. B. Romero-Moraleda et al., "Effects of Vibration and Non-vibration Foam Rolling on Recovery after Exercise with Induced Muscle Damage," *Journal of Sports Science and Medicine* 18, no. 1 (2019): 172–80, https://www.ncbi.nlm.nih.gov/pmc/articles/PMC6370959/ (5 March 2023).

5. Jian Chen, "Rhabdomyolysis after the Use of Percussion Massage Gun: A Case Report," *Physical Therapy* 101, no. 1 (2021), https://doi.org/10.1093/ptj/pzaa199 (5 March 2023).

CHAPTER 16. RESTORATIVE YOGA

1. José Afonso et al., "The Effectiveness of Post-exercise Stretching in Short-Term and Delayed Recovery of Strength, Range of Motion and Delayed Onset Muscle Soreness: A Systematic Review and Meta-analysis of Randomized Controlled Trials," *Frontiers in Physiology* 12 (2021), https://doi.org/10.3389/fphys.2021.677581 (5 March 2023).

CHAPTER 17. MEDITATION AND BREATHING

1. Matt Fitzgerald, *Run: The Mind-Body Method of Running by Feel* (Boulder, CO: Velo, 2010).

2. E. Luders et al., "The Underlying Anatomical Correlates of Long-Term Meditation: Larger Hippocampal and Frontal Volumes of Gray Matter," *NeuroImage* 45 (2009): 672–78.

3. Kelly McGonigal, "Your Brain on Meditation," *Yoga Journal*, August 2010, 68–70, 92–98.

4. Herbert Benson, *The Relaxation Response* (New York: HarperCollins, 2000).

5. Benson, *The Relaxation Response*, xxii.

6. Daniele Martarelli et al., "Diaphragmatic Breathing Reduces Exercise-Induced Oxidative Stress," *Evidence-Based Complementary and Alternative Medicine* (2011), https://doi.org/10.1093/ecam/nep169 (5 March 2023).

7. Benedict Herhaus, Rupert Conrad, and Katja Petrowski, "Effect of a Slow-Paced Breathing with Heart Rate Variability Biofeedback Intervention on Pro-inflammatory Cytokines in Individuals with Panic Disorder: A Randomized Controlled Trial," *Journal of Affective Disorders* 326 (2023): 132–38, https://doi.org/10.1016/j.jad.2023.01.091 (5 March 2023).

References and Further Reading

Afonso, José, et al. "The Effectiveness of Post-exercise Stretching in Short-Term and Delayed Recovery of Strength, Range of Motion and Delayed Onset Muscle Soreness: A Systematic Review and Meta-analysis of Randomized Controlled Trials." *Frontiers in Physiology* 12 (2021). https://doi.org/10.3389/fphys.2021.677581 (5 March 2023).

Ali, A., M. P. Caine, and B. G. Snow. "Graduated Compression Stockings: Physiological and Perceptual Responses during and after Exercise." *Journal of Sports Sciences* 25 (2007): 413–19.

Anderson, Scott A., Kristin Haraldsdottir, and Drew Watson. "Mindfulness in Athletes." *Current Sports Medicine Reports* 20, no. 12 (2021): 655–60. https://journals.lww.com/acsm-csmr/Fulltext/2021/12000/Mindfulness_in_Athletes.8.aspx (5 March 2023).

Angelopoulos, P., et al. "Cold-Water Immersion and Sports Massage Can Improve Pain Sensation but Not Functionality in Athletes with Delayed Onset Muscle Soreness." *Healthcare* (Basel, Switzerland) 10, no. 12 (2022). https://doi.org/10.3390/healthcare10122449 (4 March 2023).

Apor, P., M. Petrekanich, and J. Számado. "Heart Rate Variability Analysis in Sports." *Orv Hetil* 150 (2009): 847–53.

Archer, Pat. *Therapeutic Massage in Athletics.* Baltimore: Lippincott, Williams, and Wilkins, 2007.

Armstrong, S. A., et al. "Compression Socks and Functional Recovery Following Marathon Running: A Randomized Controlled Trial." *Journal of Strength and Conditioning Research* 29, no. 2 (2015): 528–33. https://doi.org/10.1519/JSC.0000000000000649 (4 March 2023).

Baldari, C., et al. "Blood Lactate Removal during Recovery at Various Intensities Below the Individual Anaerobic Threshold in Triathletes." *Journal of Sports Medicine and Physical Fitness* 45 (2005): 460–66.

Banister, E. W. "Modeling Elite Athletic Performance." In *Physiological Testing of the High-Performance Athlete*, 2nd ed., edited by J. D. MacDougall, H. A. Wenger, and H. J. Green, 403–24. Champaign, IL: Human Kinetics, 1991.

Barber, D., et al. "Halotherapy for Chronic Respiratory Disorders: From the Cave to the Clinical." *Alternative Therapies in Health and Medicine* 28, no. 3 (2022): 52–56. https://pubmed.ncbi.nlm.nih.gov/32827399/ (4 March 2023).

Barnett, Anthony. "Using Recovery Modalities between Training Sessions in Elite Athletes: Does It Help?" *Sports Medicine* 36 (2006): 781–96.

Benson, Herbert. *The Relaxation Response.* New York: HarperCollins, 2000.

Best, T. M., et al. "Effectiveness of Sports Massage for Recovery of Skeletal Muscle from Strenuous Exercise." *Clinical Journal of Sports Medicine* 18 (2008): 446–60.

Bompa, T. O., and G. G. Haff. *Periodization.* 5th ed. Champaign, IL: Human Kinetics, 2009.

Broatch, J. R., A. Petersen, and D. J. Bishop. "Postexercise Cold Water Immersion Benefits Are Not Greater Than the Placebo Effect." *Medicine and Science in Sports and Exercise* 46, no. 11 (2014): 2139–47. https://doi.org/10.1249/MSS.0000000000000348 (4 March 2023).

Broderick, Vipan, Liis Uiga, and Matthew Driller. "Flotation-Restricted Environmental Stimulation Therapy Improves Sleep and Performance Recovery in Athletes." *Performance Enhancement and Health* 7, no. 1–2 (2019). https://doi.org/10.1016/j.peh.2019.100149 (4 March 2023).

Burr, J. F., et al. "Cannabis and Athletic Performance." *Sports Medicine* 51, suppl. 1 (2021): 75–87. https://doi.org/10.1007/s40279-021-01505-x (4 March 2023).

Chen, Jian. "Rhabdomyolysis after the Use of Percussion Massage Gun: A Case Report." *Physical Therapy* 101, no. 1 (2021). https://doi.org/10.1093/ptj/pzaa199 (5 March 2023).

Cooper, Kenneth. *The New Aerobics.* Eldora, IA: Prairie Wind, 1970.

Davies, V., K. G. Thompson, and S.-M. Cooper. "The Effects of Compression Garments on Recovery." *Journal of Strength and Conditioning Research* 23 (2009): 1786–94.

Draganich, C., and K. Erdal. "Placebo Sleep Affects Cognitive Functioning." *Journal of Experimental Psychology: Learning, Memory, and Cognition* 40, no. 3 (2014): 857–64. https://doi.org/10.1037/a0035546 (4 March 2023).

Driller, Matthew W., et al. "Pyjamas, Polysomnography, and Professional Athletes: The Role of Sleep Tracking Technology in Sport." *Sports* 11, no. 1 (2023): 14. https://doi.org/10.3390/sports11010014 (4 March 2023).

Dueck, C. A., M. M. Manore, and K. S. Matt. "Role of Energy Balance in Athletic Menstrual Dysfunction." *International Journal of Sport Nutrition and Exercise Metabolism* 6 (1996): 165–90.

Engels, H. J., M. M. Fahlman, and J. C. Wirth. "Effects of Ginseng on Secretory IgA, Performance, and Recovery from Interval Exercise." *Medicine and Science in Sports and Exercise* 35 (2003): 690–96.

Ferreira, R. M., P. N. Martins, and R. S. Goncalves. "Effects of Self-Myofascial Release Instruments on Performance and Recovery: An Umbrella Review." *International Journal of Exercise Science* 15, no. 3 (2022): 861–83. https://www.ncbi.nlm.nih.gov/pmc/articles/PMC9362891/ (5 March 2023).

Fitzgerald, Matt. *Run: The Mind-Body Method of Running by Feel.* Boulder, CO: Velo, 2010.

Foster, Carl. "Monitoring Training in Athletes with Reference to Overtraining Syndrome." *Medicine and Science in Sports and Exercise* 30 (1998): 1164–68.

Friel, Joe. *The Triathlete's Training Bible*. 3rd ed. Boulder, CO: Velo, 2009.

Friel, Joe, and Gordon Byrn. *Going Long: Training for Triathlon's Ultimate Challenge*. 2nd ed. Boulder, CO: Velo, 2009.

Gavriloff, Dimitri, et al. "Sham Sleep Feedback Delivered via Actigraphy Biases Daytime Symptom Reports in People with Insomnia: Implications for Insomnia Disorder and Wearable Devices." *Journal of Sleep Research* 27, no. 6 (2018): e12726. https://onlinelibrary.wiley.com/doi/abs/10.1111/jsr.12726 (4 March 2023).

Gill, N. D., C. M. Beaven, and C. Cook. "Effectiveness of Post-match Recovery Strategies in Rugby Players." *British Journal of Sports Medicine* 40 (2006): 260–63.

Gnacinski, S. L., B. B. Meyer, and C. A. Wahl. "Psychometric Properties of the RESTQ-Sport-36 in a Collegiate Student-Athlete Population." *Frontiers in Psychology* 12 (2021). https://doi.org/10.3389/fpsyg.2021.671919 (20 March 2023).

Greco, Viviana, et al. "Wearing an Eye Mask during Overnight Sleep Improves Episodic Learning and Alertness." *Sleep* (2022). https://doi.org/10.1093/sleep/zsac305 (4 March 2023).

Grunovas, A., et al. "Peripheral and Systemic Circulation after Local Dynamic Exercise and Recovery Using Passive Foot Movement and Electrostimulation." *Journal of Sports Medicine and Physical Fitness* 47 (2007): 335–43.

Hamblin, M. R. "Mechanisms and Mitochondrial Redox Signaling in Photobiomodulation." *Photochemistry and Photobiology* 94, no. 2 (2018): 199–212. https://doi.org/10.1111/php.12864 (4 March 2023).

Hedley, A. M., M. Climstein, and R. Hansen. "The Effects of Acute Heat Exposure on Muscular Strength, Muscular Endurance, and Muscular Power in the Euhydrated Athlete." *Journal of Strength and Conditioning Research* 16 (2002): 353–58.

Hemmings, B., et al. "Effects of Massage on Physiological Restoration, Perceived Recovery, and Repeated Sports Performance." *British Journal of Sports Medicine* 34 (2000): 113.

Herhaus, Benedict, Rupert Conrad, and Katja Petrowski. "Effect of a Slow-Paced Breathing with Heart Rate Variability Biofeedback Intervention on Pro-inflammatory Cytokines in Individuals with Panic Disorder: A Randomized Controlled Trial." *Journal of Affective Disorders* 326 (2023): 132–38. https://doi.org/10.1016/j.jad.2023.01.091 (5 March 2023).

Howatson, G., et al. "Influence of Tart Cherry Juice on Indices of Recovery Following Marathon Running." *Scandinavian Journal of Medicine and Science in Sports* 20, no. 6 (2010): 843–52.

Hyldahl, Robert D., and Jonathan M. Peake. "Combining Cooling or Heating Applications with Exercise Training to Enhance Performance and Muscle Adaptations." *Journal of Applied Physiology* 129, no. 2 (2020): 353–65.

Ingraham, Paul. "Does Epsom Salt Work? The Science and Mythology of Epsom Salt Bathing for Recovery from Muscle Pain, Soreness, or Injury." *Pain Science* online, 25 December 2021. https://www.painscience.com /articles/epsom-salts.php (5 March 2023).

Ivy, J. L., et al. "Muscle Glycogen Synthesis after Exercise: Effect of Time of Carbohydrate Ingestion." *Journal of Applied Physiology* 64 (1988): 1480–85.

Karp, J. R., et al. "Chocolate Milk as a Post-exercise Recovery Aid." *International Journal of Sport Nutrition and Exercise Metabolism* 16 (2006): 78–91.

Kauppinen, K. "Sauna, Shower, and Ice Water Immersion: Physiological Responses to Brief Exposures to Heat, Cool, and Cold, Part I: Body Fluid Balance." *Arctic Medical Research* 48 (1989): 55–63.

Kellmann, M. *Enhancing Recovery: Preventing Underperformance in Athletes.* Champaign, IL: Human Kinetics, 2002.

Kellmann, M., and K. Wolfgang Kallus. *Recovery-Stress Questionnaire for Athletes: User Manual.* Champaign, IL: Human Kinetics, 2001.

Kellmann, M., Tom Patrick, Cal Botterill, and Clare Wilson. "The Recovery-Cue and Its Use in Applied Settings: Practical Suggestions Regarding Assessment and Monitoring of Recovery." In *Enhancing Recovery: Preventing Underperformance in Athletes*, edited by M. Kellmann, 219–29. Champaign, IL: Human Kinetics, 2002.

Kemmler, W., et al. "Effect of Compression Stocking on Running Performance in Men Runners." *Journal of Strength and Conditioning Research* 23 (2009): 101–5.

Kerksick, C. M. S., et al. "International Society of Sports Nutrition Position Stand: Nutrient Timing." *Journal of the International Society of Sports Nutrition* 14, no. 1 (2017). https://doi.org/10.1186/s12970-017-0189-4 (4 March 2023).

Kirby, N. V., et al. "Intermittent Post-exercise Sauna Bathing Improves Markers of Exercise Capacity in Hot and Temperate Conditions in Trained Middle-Distance Runners." *European Journal of Applied Physiology* 121 (2021): 621–35. https://doi.org/10.1007/s00421-020-04541-z (4 March 2023).

Krueger, Malte, et al. "Whole-Body Cryotherapy (−110 °C) Following High-Intensity Intermittent Exercise Does Not Alter Hormonal, Inflammatory, or Muscle Damage Biomarkers in Trained Males." *Cytokine* 113 (2019): 277–84. https://doi.org/10.1016/j.cyto.2018.07.018 (4 March 2023).

Kuehl, K. S., et al. "Efficacy of Tart Cherry Juice in Reducing Muscle Pain during Running: A Randomized Controlled Trial." *Journal of the International Society of Sports Nutrition* 7 (2010): 17.

Lamberg, L. "Sleep May Be Athletes' Best Performance Booster." *Psychiatric News*, 19 August 2005. https://doi.org/10.1176/pn.40.16.00400021 (5 March 2023).

Lawrence, D., and V. V. Kakkar. "Graduated, Static, External Compression of the Lower Limb: A Physiological Assessment." *British Journal of Surgery* 67 (1980): 119–21.

Luders, E., et al. "The Underlying Anatomical Correlates of Long-Term Meditation: Larger Hippocampal and Frontal Volumes of Gray Matter." *NeuroImage* 45 (2009): 672–78.

MacDonald, Graham, et al. "Foam Rolling as a Recovery Tool after an Intense Bout of Physical Activity." *Medicine and Science in Sports and Exercise* 46, no. 1 (2014): 131–42. https://journals.lww.com/acsm-msse

/Fulltext/2014/01000/Foam_Rolling_as_a_Recovery_Tool_after_an
_Intense.19.aspx (5 March 2023).

Mah, C. D., et al. "The Effects of Sleep Extension on the Athletic Performance
of Collegiate Basketball Players." *Sleep* 34, no. 7 (2011): 943–50. https://doi
.org/10.5665/SLEEP.1132 (4 March 2023).

Mancinelli, C. A., et al. "The Effects of Massage on Delayed Onset Muscle
Soreness and Physical Performance in Female Collegiate Athletes." *Physical
Therapy in Sport* 7 (2006): 5–13.

Martarelli, Daniele, et al. "Diaphragmatic Breathing Reduces Exercise-
Induced Oxidative Stress." *Evidence-Based Complementary and Alternative
Medicine* (2011). https://doi.org/10.1093/ecam/nep169 (5 March 2023).

McGonigal, Kelly. "Your Brain on Meditation." *Yoga Journal*, August 2010,
68–70, 92–98.

McNair, D., M. Lorr, and L. F. Droppleman. *Profile of Mood States Manual.*
San Diego: Educational and Industrial Testing Service, 1971, 1992.

Meeusen, R., et al. "Diagnosing Overtraining in Athletes using the Two-Bout
Exercise Protocol." *British Journal of Sports Medicine* 44, no. 9 (2010): 642–
48. https://doi.org/10.1136/bjsm.2008.049981 (5 March 2023).

Mero, A., et al. "Effects of Far-Infrared Sauna Bathing on Recovery from
Strength and Endurance Training Sessions in Men." *SpringerPlus* 4 (2015).
https://doi.org/10.1186/s40064-015-1093-5 (4 March 2023).

Mesas, A. E., et al. "Is Daytime Napping an Effective Strategy to Improve
Sport-Related Cognitive and Physical Performance and Reduce Fatigue? A
Systematic Review and Meta-analysis of Randomised Controlled Trials."
British Journal of Sports Medicine online, 23 January 2023. https://bjsm.bmj
.com/content/early/2023/01/22/bjsports-2022-106355 (4 March 2023).

Negro, M., et al. "Branched-Chain Amino Acid Supplementation Does Not
Enhance Athletic Performance but Affects Muscle Recovery and the Immune
System." *Journal of Sports Medicine and Physical Fitness* 48 (2008): 347–51.

Neric, F. B., et al. "Comparison of Swim Recovery and Muscle Stimulation
on Lactate Removal after Sprint Swimming." *Journal of Strength and
Conditioning Research* 23 (2009): 2560–67.

Neubauer, O., et al. "Antioxidant Responses to an Acute Ultra-endurance Exercise: Impact on DNA Stability and Indications for an Increased Need for Nutritive Antioxidants in the Early Recovery Phase." *British Journal of Nutrition* 104 (2010): 1129–38.

Nieman, D. C., et al. "N-3 Polyunsaturated Fatty Acids Do Not Alter Immune and Inflammation Measures in Endurance Athletes." *International Journal of Sports Nutrition and Exercise Metabolism* 19 (2009): 536–46.

Poindexter, R. H., E. F. Wright, and D. F. Murchison. "Comparison of Moist and Dry Heat Penetration through Orofacial Tissues." *Cranio* 20 (2002): 28–33.

Pollan, Michael. *In Defense of Food.* New York: Penguin, 2008.

Poppendieck, W., et al. "Massage and Performance Recovery: A Meta-analytical Review." *Sports Medicine* 46 (2016): 183–204. https://doi.org/10.1007/s40279-015-0420-x (5 March 2023).

Rahman, Shadab A., et al. "Manipulating Sleep Duration Perception Changes Cognitive Performance: An Exploratory Analysis." *Journal of Psychosomatic Research* 132 (2020). https://doi.org/10.1016/j.jpsychores.2020.109992 (4 March 2023).

Ray, Melinda L., et al. "Effect of Sodium in a Rehydration Beverage When Consumed as a Fluid or Meal." *Journal of Applied Physiology* 85, no. 4 (1998): 1329–36. https://doi.org/10.1152/jappl.1998.85.4.1329 (4 March 2023).

Romero-Moraleda, B., et al. "Effects of Vibration and Non-vibration Foam Rolling on Recovery after Exercise with Induced Muscle Damage." *Journal of Sports Science and Medicine* 18, no. 1 (2019): 172–80. https://www.ncbi.nlm.nih.gov/pmc/articles/PMC6370959/ (5 March 2023).

Rountree, Sage. *The Athlete's Guide to Yoga: An Integrated Approach to Strength, Flexibility, and Focus.* Boulder, CO: Velo, 2008.

———. *The Athlete's Pocket Guide to Yoga: 50 Routines for Strength, Flexibility, and Balance.* Boulder, CO: Velo, 2009.

Rowbottom, D. G., D. Keast, and A. R. Morton. "The Emerging Role of Glutamine as an Indicator of Exercise Stress and Overtraining." *Sports Medicine* 21, no. 2 (1996): 80–97.

Rowlands, D. S., and D. P. Wadsworth. "Effect of High-Protein Feeding on Performance and Nitrogen Balance in Female Cyclists." *Medicine and Science in Sport and Exercise* 43, no. 1 (January 2011): 44–53. https://doi .org/10.1249/MSS.0b013e3181e93316.

Rusko, Heikki, ed. *Cross Country Skiing.* Malden, MA: Wiley Blackwell, 2003.

Ryan, Monique. *Sports Nutrition for Endurance Athletes.* Boulder, CO: Velo, 2007.

Samuels, Charles. "Sleep, Recovery, and Performance: The New Frontier in High-Performance Athletics." *Physical Medicine and Rehabilitation Clinics of North America* 20, no. 1 (2009): 149–59. https://doi.org/10.1016 /j.pmr.2008.10.009 (5 March 2023).

Scoon, Guy S. M., et al. "Effect of Post-exercise Sauna Bathing on the Endurance Performance of Competitive Male Runners." *Journal of Science and Medicine in Sport* 10, no. 4 (2007): 259–62. https://doi.org/10.1016 /j.jsams.2006.06.009 (4 March 2023).

Seebohar, Bob. *Nutrition Periodization for Endurance Athletes.* Boulder, CO: Bull, 2004.

Sellwood, K. L., et al. "Ice-Water Immersion and Delayed-Onset Muscle Soreness: A Randomized Controlled Trial." *British Journal of Sports Medicine* 41 (2007): 392–97.

Smith, D. J., and S. R. Norris. "Training Load and Monitoring in Athlete's Tolerance for Endurance Training." In *Enhancing Recovery: Preventing Underperformance in Athletes,* edited by M. Kellmann, 81–101. Champaign, IL: Human Kinetics, 2002.

Snyder, A. C., et al. "A Physiological/Psychological Indicator of Over-Reaching during Intensive Training." *International Journal of Sports Medicine* 14 (1993): 29–32.

Sperlich, B., et al. "Different Types of Compression Clothing Do Not Increase Sub-maximal and Maximal Endurance Performance in Well-Trained Athletes." *Journal of Sports Sciences* 28, no. 6 (2010): 609–14. https:// doi.org/10.1080/02640410903582768 (5 March 2023).

Spiegel, K., R. Leproult, and E. Van Cauter. "Impact of Sleep Debt on Metabolic and Endocrine Function." *Lancet* 354 (1999): 1435–39.

Stacey, D. L., et al. "Effects of Recovery Method after Exercise on Performance, Immune Changes, and Psychological Outcomes." *Journal of Orthopaedic and Sports Physical Therapy* 40, no. 10 (2010): 656–65. https:// doi.org/10.2519/jospt.2010.3224 (5 March 2023).

Steinacker, J. M., and M. Lehmann. "Clinical Findings and Mechanisms of Stress and Recovery in Athletes." In *Enhancing Recovery: Preventing Underperformance in Athletes*, edited by M. Kellmann, 103–18. Champaign, IL: Human Kinetics, 2002.

Struijs, Peter, and Gino Kerkhoffs. "Ankle Sprain." *British Medical Journal of Clinical Evidence* 13 (2010): 1115.

Stults-Kolehmainen, M. A., and J. B. Bartholomew. "Psychological Stress Impairs Short-Term Muscular Recovery from Resistance Exercise." *Medicine and Science in Sports and Exercise* 44, no. 11 (2012): 2220–27. https://doi.org/10.1249/MSS.0b013e31825f67a0 (5 March 2023).

Terblanche, Elmarie, and Marlize Coetzee. "The Effect of Graded Compression Socks on Maximal Exercise Capacity and Recovery in Runners." *Medicine and Science in Sports and Exercise* 39, no. 5 (2007): S350. https://doi.org/10.1249/01.mss.0000274369.11864.4b (5 March 2023).

Tessitore, A., et al. "Effectiveness of Active versus Passive Recovery Strategies after Futsal Games." *Journal of Strength and Conditioning Research* 22 (2008): 1402–12.

Thomas, Travis, Kelly Anne Erdman, and Louise M. Burke. "Position of the Academy of Nutrition and Dietetics, Dietitians of Canada, and the American College of Sports Medicine: Nutrition and Athletic Performance." *Academy Position Paper* 116, no. 3 (2016): 501–28. https://doi.org/10.1016/j.jand.2015.12.006 (5 March 2023).

Tiller, Nicholas B. *The Skeptic's Guide to Sports Science: Confronting Myths of the Health and Fitness Industry.* New York: Routledge, 2020.

Tucker, Ross, Jonathan Dugas, and Matt Fitzgerald. *The Runner's Body.* New York: Rodale, 2009.

Warden, S. J. "Prophylactic Use of NSAIDs by Athletes: A Risk/Benefit Assessment." *Physician and Sports Medicine* 38 (2010): 132–38.

Weerapong, P., P. A. Hume, and G. S. Kolt. "The Mechanisms of Massage and Effects on Performance, Muscle Recovery, and Injury Prevention." *Sports Medicine* 35 (2005): 235–56.

Wiewelhove, T., et al. "A Meta-analysis of the Effects of Foam Rolling on Performance and Recovery." *Frontiers in Physiology* 10 (2019): 376. https://doi.org/10.3389/fphys.2019.00376 (5 March 2023).

Wigernaes, I., et al. "Active Recovery Reduces the Decrease in Circulating White Blood Cells after Exercise." *International Journal of Sports Medicine* 21 (2000): 608–12.

Wilkin, L. D., et al. "Influence of Therapeutic Ultrasound on Skeletal Muscle Regeneration Following Blunt Contusion." *International Journal of Sports Medicine* 25 (2004): 73–77.

Wilson, M. G., et al. "Cardiorespiratory Considerations for Return-to-Play in Elite Athletes after COVID-19 Infection: A Practical Guide for Sport and Exercise Medicine Physicians." *British Journal of Sports Medicine* 54 (2020): 1157–61. https://bjsm.bmj.com/content/54/19/1157 (4 March 2023).

Wiltshire, E. V., et al. "Massage Impairs Postexercise Muscle Blood Flow and 'Lactic Acid' Removal." *Medicine and Science in Sports and Exercise* 42 (2010): 1062–71.

Index

About the Author

Sage Rountree (sagerountree.com), PhD, is a specialist in yoga for athletes, an endurance sports coach, a yoga teacher trainer at the highest level (E-RYT 500), and co-owner of the Carolina Yoga Company and Hillsborough Spa and Day Retreat. She has been a regular contributor to *Yoga Journal* and *Runner's World*, where she sat on the advisory board from 2008 to 2018.

Rountree spent more than 10 years as the private yoga teacher for Naismith Memorial Basketball Hall of Fame coach Roy Williams. She has worked extensively with the University of North Carolina football, men's basketball, men's lacrosse, and cross-country teams. She has also taught the Charlotte Hornets as a team, as well as many individual NBA and NFL players.

In her 10-plus years of coaching, Rountree led athletes to peak performances in races including the World Duathlon Championships, the Ironman 70.3 World Championship, the Leadville 100 MTB race, and running races of distances from 5K to 100 miles. She has personally competed at a variety of distances, running races from 400 meters to 40 miles and finishing triathlons of every distance from super sprint to Ironman. She represented Team USA at the 2008 Age-Group World Triathlon Championships in Vancouver, Canada.

Rountree's numerous other books include *Racing Wisely: A Practical and Philosophical Guide to Performing at Your Personal Best* (2013), *Everyday Yoga: At-Home Routines to Enhance Fitness, Build Strength, and Restore Your Body* (2015), *Lifelong Yoga: Maximizing Your Balance, Flexibility, and Core Strength in Your 50s, 60s, and Beyond* (2017, cowritten with Alexandra DeSiato), and *The Professional Yoga Teacher's Handbook* (2020). She lives with her husband, Wes, in North Carolina.